Restless Legs Syndrome

AMERICAN ACADEMY OF NEUROLOGY (AAN)
Quality of Life Guides
Lisa M. Shulman, MD
Series Editor

Alzheimer's Disease
Paul Dash, MD and Nicole Villemarette-Pittman, PhD

Amyotrophic Lateral Sclerosis
Robert G. Miller, MD, Deborah Gelinas, MD,
and Patricia O'Connor, RN

Epilepsy
Ilo E. Leppik, MD

Guillain-Barré Syndrome
Gareth John Parry, MD and Joel Steinberg, MD

Migraine and Other Headaches
William B. Young, MD and Stephen D. Silberstein, MD

Peripheral Neuropathy
Norman Latov, MD

Restless Legs Syndrome
Mark J. Buchfuhrer, MD, Wayne A. Hening, MD, PhD,
and Clete Kushida, MD, PhD

Stroke
Louis R. Caplan, MD

Understanding Pain
Harry J. Gould, III, MD, PhD

Restless Legs Syndrome
Coping with Your Sleepless Nights

MARK J. BUCHFUHRER, MD, FRCP(C), FCCP
Director
SomnoMedix Sleep Disorders Center
Lakewood, California

WAYNE A. HENING, MD, PhD
Assistant Clinical Professor of Neurology
UMDNJ-RW Johnson Medical School
New Brunswick, New Jersey

CLETE A. KUSHIDA, MD, PhD
Director
Stanford University Center for Human Sleep Research
Associate Professor
Stanford University Medical Center
Palo Alto, California

With contributions from
Ann. E. Battenfield, CPT, MA Instructional Design
Karla M. Dzienkowski, RN, BSN

LISA M. SHULMAN, MD
Series Editor
Associate Professor of Neurology
Rosalyn Newman Distinguished Scholar in Parkinson's Disease
Co-Director, Maryland Parkinson's Disease
and Movement Disorders Center
University of Maryland School of Medicine
Baltimore, Maryland

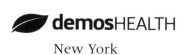

New York

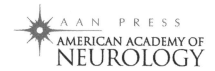

Library of Congress Cataloging-in-Publication Data

Buchfuhrer, Mark J.
  Restless legs syndrome : coping with your sleepless nights / Mark J. Buchfuhrer, Wayne A. Hening, Clete A. Kushida ; with contributions from Ann. E. Battenfield, Karla M. Dzienkowski.
      p. cm. — (American Academy of Neurology (AAN) quality of life guides)
  Includes bibliographical references and index.
  ISBN-13: 978-1-932603-57-6 (pbk. : alk. paper)
  ISBN-10: 1-932603-57-3 (pbk. : alk. paper)
  1. Restless legs syndrome. I. Hening, Wayne A. II. Kushida, Clete Anthony, 1960– III. Battenfield, Ann. E. IV. Dzienkowski, Karla M. V. Title.
  RC548.5.B83 2007
  616.8'4—dc22

                                                                                    2006026768

Medicine is an ever-changing science undergoing continual development. Research and clinical experience are continually expanding our knowledge, in particular our knowledge of proper treatment and drug therapy. The authors, editors, and publisher have made every effort to ensure that all information in this book is in accordance with the state of knowledge at the time of production of the book.

Nevertheless, this does not imply or express any guarantee or responsibility on the part of the authors, editors, or publisher with respect to any dosage instructions and forms of application stated in the book. Every reader should examine carefully the package inserts accompanying each drug and check with a his physician or specialist whether the dosage schedules mentioned therein or the contraindications stated by the manufacturer differ from the statements made in this book. Such examination is particularly important with drugs that are either rarely used or have been newly released on the market. Every dosage schedule or every form of application used is entirely at the reader's own risk and responsibility. The editors and publisher welcome any reader to report to the publisher any discrepancies or inaccuracies noticed.

Special discounts on bulk quantities of Demos Medical Publishing books are available to corporations, professional associations, pharmaceutical companies, health care organizations and other qualifying groups. For details, please contact:

Special Sales Department
Demos Medical Publishing
11 W. 42nd Street
New York, NY 10036
Phone: (800) 532-8663; (212) 683-0072
Fax: 212-941-7842
Email ordering: rsantana@demosmedpub.com

Made in the United States of America

This book is dedicated to Orren Hawley, Virginia Wilson, and Pickett Guthrie, who brought the Restless Legs Syndrome Foundation into being, and to Arthur Walter, who first realized that patients and physicians should work together to bring relief to the millions of RLS sufferers.

I would also like to dedicate this book to my mother and father, Rose and Norbert Buchfuhrer, holocaust survivors who passed on the determination and dedication necessary to write and edit this book on RLS.

Contents

About the AAN Press
Quality of Life Guides

IN THE SPIRIT OF THE DOCTOR-PATIENT PARTNERSHIP

THE BETTER-INFORMED PATIENT is often able to play a vital role in his or her own care. This is especially the case with neurologic disorders, for which effective management of disease can be promoted—indeed, *enhanced*—through patient education and involvement.

In the spirit of the partnership-in-care between physicians and patients, the American Academy of Neurology Press is pleased to produce a series of "Quality of Life" guides on an array of diseases and ailments that affect the brain and central nervous system. The series, produced in partnership with Demos Medical Publishing, answers a number of basic and important questions faced by patients and their families.

Additionally, the authors, most of whom are physicians and all of whom are experts in the areas in which they write, provide a detailed discussion of the disorder, its causes, and the course it may follow. You also find strategies for coping with the disorder and handling a number of nonmedical issues.

The result: As a reader, you will be able to develop a framework for understanding the disease and become better prepared to manage the life changes associated with it.

ABOUT THE AMERICAN ACADEMY OF NEUROLOGY (AAN)

The American Academy of Neurology is the premier organization for neurologists worldwide. In addition to support of educational and scientific advances, the AAN—along with its sister organization, the AAN Foundation—is a strong advocate of public education and a leading supporter of research for breakthroughs in neurologic patient care.

More information on the activities of the AAN is available on our website, www.aan.com. For a better understanding of common disorders of the brain, as well as to learn about people living with these disorders, please turn to the AAN Foundation's website, www.thebrainmatters.org.

About Neurology and Neurologists

Neurology is the medical specialty associated with disorders of the brain and central nervous system. Neurologists are medical doctors with specialized training in the diagnosis, treatment, and management of patients suffering from neurologic disease.

Lisa M. Shulman, MD
Series Editor
AAN Press Quality of Life Guides

Foreword

T OO OFTEN, THE TERM "restless legs syndrome" (RLS) generates snick- ers of amusement from anyone who is ill informed about this puz- zling condition. For years, most people with RLS suffered alone. It wasn't until 1989 that eight RLS sufferers from across the US began exchanging letters. Medical knowledge about RLS was so limited that others afflicted with the strange-sounding disorder turned to this fledg- ling support group in search of coping methods and therapies. In 1992, this coalition of sleep-deprived amateurs launched the Restless Legs Syndrome Foundation, a non-profit organization, dedicated to alerting the world that restless legs syndrome is real and treatable.

Their grassroots effort soon attracted the attention of a small group of sleep researchers. This team of RLS pioneers became the nucleus of the foundation's first medical advisory board and continues to lead the way in unraveling the mystery behind RLS.

Despite numerous studies estimating that as many as 10 percent of Americans have this potentially devastating disorder, RLS is still hardly a household word. Other than material published by the RLS founda- tion, people with RLS have had difficulty finding credible information about the condition. This book helps fill the need for reliable informa- tion and represents another milestone in the collaboration between patients, researchers, and clinicians. Patients and their families will appreciate the clear, concise descriptions of who gets RLS, what causes RLS, and how RLS is diagnosed. Even those who learned long ago the name of the culprit behind their sleepless nights will welcome this up- to-date review of treatment options.

Drs. Buchfuhrer, Hening, and Kushida are part of an effective part- nership between patients and medical professionals that has spearhead- ed advances in treatment and improved life for RLS sufferers. All three have served on the foundation's medical advisory board, written articles for the foundation's quarterly newsletter, and answered hundreds of questions from patients who struggle with this potentially devastating condition. Along with impressive credentials, they each have the rare ability to translate medical and scientific terms into language that is accessible to any reader.

Topics covered in this book include non-pharmacological therapies (such as alerting activities and abstaining from caffeine, nicotine and alcohol); complementary and alternative medicine (vitamins, herbal remedies, chiropractic and acupuncture); intermittent drug treatment for those with sporadic symptoms; medications for those who contend with the disruptive symptoms of restless legs on a daily basis; and the future of RLS treatment.

In keeping with their philosophy of teamwork, the authors include material from two people directly affected by the disorder. The chapter on "RLS and Relationships" is written by Ann Battenfield, herself an RLS patient and volunteer moderator for one of the RLS online discussion boards. Her section offers tips for dealing with the stress of living with the disorder. Karla Dzienkowski is the mother of a 15-year-old with RLS. She is also a registered nurse and member of the foundation's board of directors. Her chapter on "RLS in Children and Adolescents" outlines coping strategies for families dealing with the disorder in younger patients.

Fifteen years of collaboration between patients and medical professionals have improved RLS treatments and fueled rapid progress in unraveling the science that may someday lead to a cure. The authors and contributors to this book continue to prove that teamwork is the best hope for millions of men, women, and children who must live with restless legs syndrome.

Pickett M. Guthrie, MLS
Co-Founder Restless Legs Syndrome Foundation
Executive Director, 1992–1996
Member, Board of Directors, 2003–Present

Preface

"Restless Legs Syndrome: the most common disease you've never heard of."

ROBERT YOAKUM
Former Board Member
Restless Legs Syndrome Foundation

IF YOU ARE READING THIS BOOK then it is very likely that you or someone close to you has restless legs syndrome (RLS). It is also likely that you understand how well Robert Yoakum's quote typifies the lack of awareness about RLS. You have probably experienced the frustration of dealing with medical professionals, most of whom have very little knowledge about or ability to treat this disease, despite its high prevalence in the U.S. population. Until recently, RLS has been the "Rodney Dangerfield" of sleep and neurologic disorders, with little respect being given to patients or even to doctors treating or researching this trivial-sounding disease. It is common for an RLS patient to be told that the problem is "all in your head" or "doesn't exist" or that "you are just too anxious."

The RLS Foundation, which was created in 1992, has been working very hard to change this situation. This nonprofit organization provides support for RLS patients, doctors, educators, and researchers. It has been the driving force in the effort to increase awareness of this poorly known disease.

We are now at the dawn of a new age of RLS awareness and treatment. The FDA approved the first drug to treat RLS in May 2005, and several more are pending. Having an FDA-approved drug adds to the credibility of this disease. In the next few years, RLS should become much better known and gain the recognition and respect it deserves.

Although RLS is not a curable disease, its symptoms are very treatable. With proper care, most patients can achieve dramatic relief, if not complete resolution of their symptoms. RLS patients should not despair, but rather take a proactive approach to managing their disease. This book helps guide RLS patients through the often very difficult path of managing their disease successfully.

All aspects of RLS and periodic limb movement disorder (PLMD) are discussed in this book. Readers will become more familiar with the presentation, diagnosis, course, and causes of RLS and PLMD. The chapter on management of RLS and PLMD covers all aspects of treatment extensively. It reviews all of the helpful drug and nondrug therapies. After reading this book, patients should become very familiar and comfortable with the management of this disorder.

Although this book is meant for RLS sufferers all over the world, the drug treatment of this disease varies from country to country due to the different availability of these drugs. Narcotics are more freely prescribed in the U.S., while drugs such as cabergoline are used more in Europe where they are less expensive. RLS patients in some countries do not have access to the newer drugs like Mirapex and Requip, while we here in the U.S. do not have domperidone, an inexpensive antinausea drug that does not worsen RLS. Clearly, the choice of RLS therapies can differ significantly based on the availability of drugs and the prevailing attitudes of their use.

RLS sufferers should take an active role in managing their disease. We discuss how they should work with their doctors to achieve optimal therapy. This book gives guidelines for the very difficult task of finding and choosing the right doctor to treat RLS.

Patients often have difficulties coping with their RLS symptoms and the limitations resulting from this disease. We discuss many techniques for coping with the different aspects of life affected by RLS and PLMD, including daily activities, recreational activities, emotions, psychiatric problems, and medical procedures. RLS sufferers will also learn how to deal with relationships that are often strained by this chronic disease.

RLS in children is quite common but is less well known and diagnosed than in adults. The book covers this topic as well as the treatment of children. We encourage parents of children with RLS to read the section on how to cope with RLS in young children and teenagers.

We encourage all RLS patients to become more educated about their disease. The Appendix contains information on other sources to continue your education. Included are resources for educating your health care professional. We also encourage all RLS patients to join the RLS Foundation and a local support group. By doing so, you will help both yourself and other RLS sufferers.

We hope this book will help those suffering from RLS or PLMD to manage and live with their disease. They will learn not to be embarrassed by their strange-sounding symptoms. Instead of suffering quietly, patients will learn how to get proper care, which should relieve the symptoms of most RLS sufferers.

The future for RLS sufferers looks much brighter now. We expect that over the next decade RLS will become a well-known disease. Patients will no longer have to struggle to be diagnosed and treated for their disruptive symptoms. As research accelerates, more therapies should make effective treatment even more accessible. Because of the fast pace of change in our knowledge about this disease, some of the therapies discussed in this book may be quite different in the next few years.

Mark J. Buchfuhrer, MD, FRCP(C), FCCP
Wayne A. Hening, MD, PhD
Clete A. Kushida, MD, PhD

Acknowledgments

I WOULD LIKE TO THANK the Restless Legs Syndrome Foundation, its founders, board of directors, advisors, and staff members, who have worked for so many years to increase the awareness of RLS, which has resulted in the demand for this book. The RLS Foundation has been integral in educating the public and medical professionals, raising money, and spearheading research on this perplexing disorder.

I would like to thank Elizabeth "Bill" Tunison, previous RLS Foundation board member and founder of the Southern California RLS Support Group, for gently but persistently guiding me into the field of RLS.

I would like to thank the family members of all the authors who supported us during the writing of the book.

I also thank my wife, Laurie Buchfuhrer, MD, for her patience and her support and her many helpful suggestions while writing this book.

Restless Legs Syndrome

CHAPTER 1

What Are Restless Legs Syndrome and Periodic Limb Movement Disorder?

I F YOU ARE READING THIS BOOK you probably already know something about restless legs syndrome (RLS) and periodic limb movement disorder (PLMD). You may even know more than most physicians about these two common conditions. Despite being poorly known and understood, approximately 10 percent of the Caucasian population in the U.S. has RLS. There is a lot of confusion about RLS and PLMD, with many physicians and people mistaking one for the other. This misunderstanding arises because they often appear together, but in fact they are two separate and distinct disorders.

RLS is a *neurologic sleep and movement disorder* characterized by an almost irresistible urge or need to move the limbs, usually related to uncomfortable limb sensations, which are worse during inactivity. Movement of the limbs occurs in order to relieve the uncomfortable sensations. A person with RLS must be awake and conscious to be bothered by RLS. In order to relieve their RLS symptoms and fall asleep, people with RLS often move their limbs and toss and turn in bed, which may disturb their bed partners (Figure 1-1).

People who experience *periodic limb movements* (PLM) have limb muscle jerks that occur mostly when they are asleep and occasionally when they are awake. People with PLMD and their bed partners are usually able to sleep in spite of the leg movements, as long as the movements are not too vigorous. RLS is an awake sensory phenomenon with

1

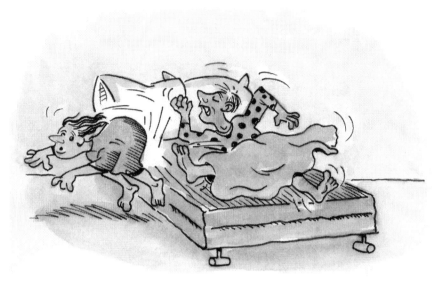

FIGURE 1-1

My wife tells me that my legs were restless again last night. She said that she didn't sleep a wink, but I slept fine.

movement due to the sensations, whereas PLM is a sleep (and only occasionally an awake) movement phenomenon that usually has no sensory component. Confusion can arise because RLS and PLM often occur together; however, they are not identical, and it must be remembered that either can exist without the other.

Despite extensive research, the cause of RLS and PLM is still unknown. The leading hypothesis at this time involves problems with dopamine function and iron in the brain. This is discussed further in Chapter 6. Although there is no cure for RLS or PLM, current therapies should relieve most people's symptoms, as discussed further in Chapter 4.

Most cases of RLS and PLM are *primary* and occur in otherwise normal healthy individuals. *Secondary* RLS and PLM occur in association with certain underlying medical conditions, as discussed in Chapter 3.

RLS = urge to move with unpleasant limb sensations occurring while awake.

RESTLESS LEGS SYNDROME

Uncomfortable Limb Sensations

Although most people with RLS have difficulty describing their uncomfortable sensations, many do not describe any abnormal sensation other than the almost irresistible urge to move the affected limb. Abnormal sensations are not necessary, however, to establish the diagnosis of RLS. The medical term for these sensations is *dysesthesia*, which is defined as a "disagreeable or abnormal sensation." Many people with RLS do not agree with the use of this term, but it is the most accurate word available to describe the sensations. RLS sufferers often describe such sensations as like ants crawling in their legs, creepy-crawly feelings, pulling sensations, water running inside their legs, or electricity in their legs. Some can only describe the sensation as an urge to move their legs. Although RLS usually starts in the legs, it can also occur in the arms or other muscles in the body as the condition progresses. Most people with RLS do not describe these sensations as painful. To better understand this, consider the analogy of how it feels to be tickled. Most of us would not describe being tickled as painful. However, if the tickling continues for too long, it can become quite bothersome and so unbearable that we might begin to consider it painful.

A minority of people experience painful symptoms, which are often described as burning, aching, or simply painful. These symptoms may occur in addition to the more typical sensations. However, in some people the painful symptoms may be the result of some separate but associated problem, such as *neuropathy* (disease of the nerves).

The large variability of the uncomfortable sensations and the difficulty in describing them contributes to problems in communicating with physicians. Many people are even reluctant to mention their symptoms because they feel they are "just too weird." Therefore, it is not surprising that physicians often miss the diagnosis of RLS. People often diagnose themselves, typically after reading a description of RLS.

What's in a Name?

Many people with RLS and their families have made up their own names for the disorder. Table 1-1 lists some of the colorful terms that people use to talk about the condition before they learn the commonly accepted name, RLS. Many people do not agree with the use of the term "restless legs syndrome," because they feel it makes the condition sound trivial, which results in physicians and others not taking it seriously.

Table 1-1   Patient's Names for RLS

Achy knees	Having butterflies in my	Racer legs
Achy legs	legs	Racing legs
Aerobic sleeping	Hopping legs	Spider legs
Alien legs	Hot legs	Spongy leg disease
Ant legs	Itchy blood	Stretchy legs
Antsy legs	Itchy chin-bone	Symphony feet
Anxious feet	Jello legs	That icky twitchy leg thing
Anxious legs	Jiggles in my legs	That knee thing
Bone itch	Jiggy legs	The crawlies
Bugs crawling in my legs at	Jimmy legs	The crawls
night	Jumpies	The creepers
Bugs in the bones	Jumpy knees	The creepy crawlies legs
Busy legs	Jumpy legs	The crinkles
Butterfly twitches	Jumpy life	The fidgits
Crawly legs	Kickies	The gotta moves
Crazy leg thing	Kicky legs	The grunions
Crazy legs	Last nerve disease	The ickies
Dancing legs	Lead legs	The itchies
Day crawls	Leaping legs	The jerks
Dead legs	Leg thrashies	The jiggies
Edgy legs	Legitis	The jitters
Eeeky	Legs are mad	The kicks
Feet cramps	Legs want to break dance	The knee jerk
Fidgety legs	Magic legs	The leggy thing
Flapping legs	Mom's leg thing	The misery
Floggin legs	Muzzy legs	The nadgers
Funny bone legs	My hands and feet are	The screeches
Funny legs	nervous	The scritchees
Grasshopper legs	Nervous leg syndrome	The shpilkes
Great RLS boogie	Night crawls	The stomps
Happy feet	Night thrashers	The tingles
Heebee-jeebees	Nighttime jitterbug	Walking legs

Groups of people with RLS have lobbied to change the name to *Ekbom's syndrome*, after Dr. Karl Ekbom, who first described RLS in 1944. Dr. Ekbom first called it *irritable legs*, but changed it to *restless legs syndrome* in 1945. Since then, the medical and scientific world has accepted and used this term, and it would be confusing to change the name again.

The Urge to Move the Affected Limb

This cardinal symptom of RLS must be present to establish the diagnosis. Many people with RLS do not have uncomfortable limb sensations, but they all have an almost irresistible urge to move the affected limb when at rest. Many people with RLS have some control over this urge and can usually delay moving for a short time as well as choose the type of movement (walking, shaking, or rubbing their leg). This is quite similar to the urge to scratch a mosquito bite. We can voluntarily stop ourselves from scratching using our willpower but, if distracted, will immediately scratch the itchy spot. However, with RLS, if the urge to move is suppressed for too long, it becomes so intense that the person loses control and must move.

Many people say they move their affected limb because it brings complete or partial relief of the uncomfortable sensations; however, the RLS symptoms and the urge to move the limb often return once the limb is at rest again. The length of time that a person can sit or lie down before feeling the urge to move decreases as RLS worsens. This can make it impossible for them to perform sedentary activities, such as watching television or going to bed and falling asleep.

Early in the disorder, the symptoms may occur only at bedtime and can be relatively mild. Once the patient is tired enough, falling asleep at bedtime may not be a problem. However, as the disorder progresses, the RLS symptoms can become intense enough that sleep is almost impossible. As the disorder progresses, symptoms usually occur earlier in the day. People with severe RLS may even have symptoms upon awakening. RLS symptoms usually start in the legs, but as the condition worsens, the symptoms move to the arms and other muscles of the body, such as the abdomen, chest, back, neck, and even the facial muscles.

How Does Your RLS Rate?

Many people with RLS wonder how their RLS problems compare with others'. Often the only reference point is a comparison to the level of RLS early in the course of the disorder. Speaking to other people with RLS may be helpful, but it may not help you define the level of your RLS within the spectrum of the disorder.

Several RLS rating scales are used to assess severity in medical studies. You can rate your RLS using the simple rating system shown in Table 1-2, which is based loosely on the validated Johns Hopkins restless legs severity scale that assigns severity based on the time of day that symptoms begin. This crude severity rating scale rates most people with RLS fairly well, but it does not take into account the intensity of the RLS symptoms and their effect on sleep and daytime functioning. It also excludes people who do not get symptoms at bedtime, but experience them only with prolonged sitting, such as on a long airplane trip.

Table 1-2	Severity of RLS
Severity	**Time of day when symptoms usually start (>50 percent of the time)**
Mild	Bedtime symptoms only
Moderate	Evening symptoms starting after 6 P.M.
Severe	Afternoon symptoms starting after 12 P.M. (noon)
Very severe	Morning symptoms

The International RLS Study Group Rating Scale

The International RLS Study Group rating scale can be used to determine a more accurate severity rating. This scale, validated in 2003, is currently considered the standard scale by most RLS specialists. To evaluate the severity of your RLS, simply answer the questions below, add up the appropriate number of points, and find your severity level in Table 1-3. Use the average symptoms you experienced during the most recent 2-week period for evaluating symptom severity.

Table 1-3   Overall Severity of RLS from IRLS Rating Scale

Severity	Total points from 10 IRLS questions
Mild	1-10
Moderate	11-20
Severe	21-30
Very severe	31-40

1. How would you rate the RLS discomfort in your legs or arms?

Very severe:	4 points
Severe:	3 points
Moderate:	2 points
Mild:	1 point
None:	0 points

2. How would you rate the need to move around because of your RLS symptoms?

Very severe:	4 points
Severe:	3 points
Moderate:	2 points
Mild:	1 point
None:	0 points

3. How much relief of your RLS arm or leg discomfort do you get from moving around?

No relief:	4 points
Slight relief:	3 points
Moderate relief:	2 points
Complete or almost complete relief:	1 point
No RLS symptoms:	0 points

4. How severe is your sleep disturbance from your RLS symptoms?

Very severe:	4 points
Severe:	3 points
Moderate:	2 points
Mild:	1 point
None:	0 points

5. How severe is your tiredness or sleepiness from your RLS symptoms?

Very severe:	4 points
Severe:	3 points
Moderate:	2 points
Mild:	1 point
None:	0 points

6. How severe is your RLS as a whole?

Very severe:	4 points
Severe:	3 points
Moderate:	2 points
Mild:	1 point
None:	0 points

7. How often do you get RLS symptoms?

Very severe (6–7 days a week):	4 points
Severe (4–5 days a week):	3 points
Moderate (2–3 days a week):	2 points
Mild (1 day a week or less):	1 point
None:	0 points

8. When you have RLS symptoms, how severe are they on an average day?

Very severe (8 hours per 24-hour day or more):	4 points
Severe (3–8 hours per 24-hour day):	3 points
Moderate (1–3 hours per 24-hour day):	2 points
Mild (less than 1 hour per 24-hour day):	1 point
None:	0 points

9. How severe is the impact of your RLS symptoms on your ability to carry out your daily affairs, for example, having a satisfactory family, home, social, school, or work life?

Very severe:	4 points
Severe:	3 points
Moderate:	2 points
Mild:	1 point
None:	0 points

10. How severe is your mood disturbance from your RLS symptoms, for example: angry, depressed, sad, anxious, or irritable?

Very severe: 4 points

Severe: 3 points

Moderate: 2 points

Mild: 1 point

None: 0 points

PLMD

What exactly is PLMD? Initially, this condition was called *nocturnal myoclonus* because the leg jerks occurred mainly at night (nocturnal) and involved contractions of a group of muscles (myoclonus). Many physicians still use this phrase, but the more current and accepted term is *periodic limb movement disorder*. Table 1-4 contains definitions of the terms related to PLMD.

PLM are the leg kicks or jerks experienced by more than 80 percent of people with RLS. However, PLM most often occurs without RLS.

PLM = limb muscle jerks mostly while asleep (PLMS).

Some people will develop RLS in the future, but most will experience only PLM and never have any RLS symptoms. The two disorders are separate and distinct entities, but they are linked in many ways. Aside from being common in people with RLS, PLM are thought to result from mechanisms similar to RLS and to respond to the same therapy.

Periodic limb movements in sleep (PLMS) are also common in other sleep disorders, including sleep apnea and narcolepsy. Some sleep specialists think that PLMS are a nonspecific response to disturbed sleep, rather than a distinct disorder. They is also more prevalent in older people who usually have no sleep complaints or problems from leg kicks. PLMS are also more common in conditions associated with secondary RLS, including pregnancy, iron-deficiency anemia, and kidney failure (see Chapter 3).

PLMS differ from the hypnic jerks, or "sleep starts," commonly experienced by normal people. These jerks are involuntary local or general

Table 1-4   Periodic Limb Movement: Acronyms and Definitions

Acronym	Definition
PLM	Periodic Limb Movement(s)—One or more leg movement in a series of rhythmic repetitive leg movements manifested by extension of the big toe, dorsiflexion of the ankle with or without flexion of the knee and hip occurring in wake or sleep. The movement can also occur in the arms. This term can also be used as the plural form for many limb movements.
PLMS	Periodic Limb Movement(s) in Sleep— One or more PLM that occur during sleep. Usually used in the plural form, referring to all the leg movements occurring during sleep or to the condition of having these leg movements during sleep.
PLMW	Periodic Limb Movement(s) during Wakefulness—One or more PLM that occur while the patient is awake. Usually used in the plural form.
PLMA	Periodic Limb Movement(s) with arousals—Leg movements that occur during sleep and result in a shift from deeper to lighter sleep.
PLMI	Periodic Limb Movement Index—Number of PLM per hour. Usually refers to the number of PLMS per each hour of sleep.
PLMAI	Periodic Limb Movement Arousal Index—Number of PLMS associated with an arousal per hour of sleep.
PLMD	Periodic Limb Movement Disorder—A medical disorder resulting from a significant frequency of PLMS during sleep with a related clinical complaint such as daytime sleepiness. The PLMS cannot be due to another disorder (sleep apnea, narcolepsy or RLS). Therefore, people with RLS cannot have PLMD.

muscle contractions that take place during the transition from wakefulness to sleep. They are often described as an electric shock or falling sensation and can cause significant body movement in bed. Stress, irregular sleep patterns, and discomfort may increase the occurrence of sleep starts. Many people confuse hypnic jerks with the leg jerks of PLMS. However, hypnic jerks occur only once or twice a night, whereas PLMS recur frequently throughout the night.

The leg kicks of PLM typically consist of a rhythmic extension of the big toe (the big toe moves upwards) and dorsiflexion of the ankle (the foot moves upwards at the ankle), with flexion at the knee and hip. Flexion at the knee and hip, which can result in vigorous leg kicks, only occurs occasionally. People vary considerably in how their leg muscles jerk, with most having unnoticeable contractions. The movements last from 1/2 second up to 10 seconds and occur about every 20–40 seconds, although there may be intervals of 5–90 seconds. They can occur in one leg at a time or both legs simultaneously. At times, the arms may also be involved.

PLM follow a *circadian* (24-hour, or daily) rhythm identical to that of RLS symptoms. They increase during the evening and night and improve in the morning. PLM occur more frequently in NREM (non–rapid eye movement, or nondreaming) sleep during the first half of the sleep period. Although typically these leg kicks are noticed by bed partners, a sleep study in which the leg muscles are monitored with (EMG) electromyography electrodes and the brain waves are monitored by EEG (electroencephalogram, or brain wave) electrodes is necessary to diagnose the extent of PLMS and whether they cause arousals.

The term PLMD is used only when PLM cause significant enough problems to result in a recognized medical disorder; however, whether or not PLMD is a *real* disorder is still quite controversial. Many sleep specialists do not believe that PLMS—even when associated with arousals—can cause a significant enough sleep disturbance to decrease the patient's daytime alertness. There is insufficient evidence to prove definitively that frequent leg kicks (with or without arousals) cause a real disorder that would warrant the term PLMD. Many sleep specialists, however, believe that PLMD does exist and should be treated.

All sleep specialists agree that the term PLMD should not be used if there are only a few leg kicks and they do not cause any sleep disruption. As discussed above, these leg kicks are called PLMS when they occur during sleep and *periodic limb movements during wakefulness* (PLMW) when they occur while awake.

Many people notice that their bed partner kicks occasionally, and they may be concerned that their bed partner might have PLMD. However, a few leg kicks do not necessarily confirm a diagnosis of PLMD. For true PLMD to exist there must be more than five PLM per hour for children and more than 15 per hour for adults. In addition, the movements must disturb the patients' sleep sufficiently to affect their ability to stay awake during the day. A sleep study to record even the minutest of leg muscle contractions is necessary to quantify the PLM, because many of the leg jerks may be minimal and imperceptible to an observer. In addition, the sleep study can count the number of PLM that cause arousals (brief awakenings from sleep) and thus prevent deep, restorative sleep.

Most people experience weak leg muscle contractions that are hardly apparent and may not bother the patients or their bed partners. The movements may consist of only a raised toe or foot. These people do not know they have PLM except when monitored in a sleep lab that can record these barely perceptible leg muscle contractions. However, the leg jerks can be violent enough to kick a patient's bed partner out of bed or break the patient's toe—luckily, these are rare events. PLM can also cause leg muscle soreness the next day. People with PLMS have complained of getting up in the morning feeling as if they have been vigorously exercising all night.

It is most common for these movements to occur while the patient is asleep (PLMS). They can also occur when awake, especially when sitting in the evening or while in bed trying to get to sleep. This is an example of PLMW. We can also divide the problems caused by PLM into two groups: those that disturb the patient and those that disturb the bed partner.

PLM That Disturb the Bed Partner, but Not the Person Who Kicks

Most people with PLM produce few arousals and may have no problem with their nighttime kicks other than the complaints of their bed partners. Most people are not aware that they are kicking at night. Like those who snore loudly and vehemently deny it (even after hearing a tape recording of their snoring), people with PLM will also deny their nightly kicking. People with PLM may not retain any conscious memory of it because the movements occur while they are asleep. PLM are usually noticed first by bed partners, who complain about being kicked and may even have bruises to prove it.

The bed partner's complaint of being kicked is often the main reason for seeking medical help, because maintaining harmony in a relationship that is affected by nighttime kicking can be an important issue. Many people with PLM that only bother their bed partners' sleep will

> The bed partner's complaint of being kicked is often the main reason for seeking medical help for PLMS, because maintaining harmony in a relationship that is disrupted by nighttime kicking can be an important issue.

demand medication so they can continue to sleep with their partners. However, physicians usually do not like to use medications to treat problems not directly affecting the patient. Helpful nondrug solutions will be discussed in Chapter 4.

PLM That Disturb the Sleep of the Person Experiencing Them

PLM can disturb sleep in two ways. The first is by preventing the person from falling asleep or by waking the person up from sleep and then preventing further sleep. The second way is by causing frequent sleep arousals (brief awakenings from sleep), which may result in nonrestorative sleep and daytime sleepiness.

The PLM may be frequent and vigorous enough to disturb a person's sleep. If these more vigorous PLM occur while the person is still awake in bed (PLMW), they may result in insomnia. Vigorous leg kicks can also wake the person up in the middle of the night. If the kicks continue, the person may be unable to go back to sleep. Little controversy exists about treating PLM that are vigorous and frequent enough to prevent people from regularly getting to sleep or sustaining sleep. People experiencing these types of PLM usually seek medical attention.

Controversy arises with leg kicks that do not awaken the person experiencing them, but cause sleep arousals. Sleep arousals are brief awakenings from sleep that last a minimum of 3 seconds. The person will not be aware of sleep arousals because he or she is not awake and conscious when they occur. The only way to document sleep arousals is by performing a sleep study with EMG electrode monitoring of the legs, which can record minimal leg muscle contractions, and EEG electrode monitoring.

The reason for the controversy is that it has not been proven that sleep arousals from PLM really do cause daytime sleepiness. Many studies have shown that the frequent sleep arousals resulting from obstructive sleep apnea cause fatigue and excessive daytime somnolence, but this may not necessarily apply to arousals due to PLM. It is necessary to show that eliminating the arousals caused by PLM improves daytime functioning. Numerous studies have demonstrated this for sleep apnea, but not yet for PLMD. In fact, one study found no relationship between the PLM arousal index and the subjective complaint of disturbed sleep, an objective measure of daytime sleepiness, or awakening refreshed in the morning.

Thus, there is a difference of opinion among RLS specialists. Some experts believe that people with frequent PLM-related sleep arousals have a *real* disorder (PLMD); others do not believe that PLMD exists. To diagnose PLMD, most sleep specialists require one to have more than 15 PLM arousals per hour in order to explain any increased daytime sleepiness. Other causes of daytime sleepiness must be ruled out, including sleep apnea, narcolepsy, or the use of medications with a side effect of sleepiness. Once these criteria are met, many sleep specialists would agree that the patient indeed has PLMD and should be treated.

A BRIEF HISTORY OF RLS

When did RLS begin to affect humans? There are rumors that the great Roman orator Cicero was afflicted by the disorder and that an even earlier Indian sage wrote about it in one of the Hindu epics. Montaigne, the great French essayist, wrote about restlessness of the legs, which was sometimes aroused by sermons in church: ". . . so that though I was seated, I was never settled."

In the Middle Ages people with RLS may have been thought to be possessed and underwent exorcism or were burned as witches. In the early modern era, the great physician and anatomist Thomas Willis described one case that many with RLS would probably recognize:

> . . . *whilst they would indulge sleep, in their beds, immediately follow leapings up of the tendons, in their arms and legs, with cramps, and such unquietness*

and flying about of their members, that the sick can no more sleep than those on the rack.

Willis seems to be clearly on point as to many features of RLS: the leg discomfort ("cramps"), the periodic limb movement while awake ("leapings up"), the onset at night ("indulge sleep"), and the difficulty sleeping, which causes the greatest problem for many people with RLS. Was Willis describing RLS? We do not know for sure, but one supportive fact is that he was able to treat one patient with a medication drawn from a class that is still used today: laudanum, a preparation of opium. He claimed a cure from this treatment, but we do not know whether a single dose, a short course, or continued treatment was necessary to control his patient's symptoms.

As mentioned earlier, Karl Ekbom, a Swedish physician, presented an almost complete picture of RLS in 1944, noting that RLS was common and could be easily diagnosed if the physician was aware of its typical symptoms. He described restlessness and movements during sleep and the difficulties his patients had with leg discomfort if they remained seated for a sustained period of time. He noted that RLS could cause difficulties with employment, the disorder ran in families, it could be increased in pregnancy or with anemia, and it could be provoked by stomach surgery that reduced the ability of the body to absorb vitamin B_{12}. It is still worthwhile to read his writings in order to get a clear picture of the various faces of RLS. Dr. Ekbom also named the disorder. At first, he considered a proper Latin name: either *asthenia crurum paraesthetica* or, for the kind of RLS with painful symptoms, *asthenia crurum dolorosa*. After some thought he settled on the simple term the disorder is known by today.

After Ekbom, RLS assumed a small niche in the medical field, and periodically another study or paper written was about it. The next major advance came from Italy, where Drs. Lugaresi and Coccagna were helping to develop the field of sleep medicine in the 1960s. One patient, a monk, came to them complaining of difficulty sleeping and jerks in his legs. Dr. Coccagna stayed up all night to monitor the patient and heard repeated scratches of the polygraph, a device used to continuously record brain waves, breathing, and muscle contractions. He peeked in at the patient and found that every 20–30 seconds the patient's legs would move. Starting with this one patient, these physicians from Bologna discovered that many people experienced the same type of movements.

Drs. Guilleminault, Weitzman, and Coleman developed a scheme for counting the movements, which they first called *periodic movements in sleep*, then *periodic leg movements in sleep*, and most recently *periodic limb movements*. Periodic limb movements were initially thought to cause major problems by disrupting sleep, and initial treatment was aimed at reducing these movements. Sometimes little distinction was made between RLS and PLMD without RLS.

A major advance was made in the early 1980s with the discovery by Sevcet Akpinar in Turkey that medications that increase the brain's dopamine activity could benefit people with RLS. Dr. Akpinar was consulted by a colonel in the Turkish military who could not sleep at night because of leg discomfort and leg jerks. He tried many different medications and found that levodopa and pergolide, a dopamine agonist (a chemical that can substitute for the brain chemical dopamine and cause a similar action), worked quite well. He was also impressed by the benefits of narcotic painkillers. A few years later, it was discovered that anticonvulsant medications such as carbamazepine (sold in the U.S. first as Tegretol®) could also benefit people with RLS. Even earlier, sedatives such as clonazepam (Klonopin®) were found to improve the quality of sleep in people with either PLMD or RLS.

In the 1990s two organizations were founded that have had a major impact in increasing education about RLS and moving the study of RLS forward: the *RLS Foundation* (RLSF) and the *International RLS Study Group* (IRLSSG). Begun as a small group that exchanged a newsletter, the RLSF was legally established in 1992 as a nonprofit corporation by Virginia Wilson and Pickett Guthrie. The RLSF has helped increase public awareness of RLS, provided public advocacy, and sponsored medical and scientific advances.

Around the same time, Dr. Arthur Walters founded the IRLSSG, which began with a few researchers in seven or so countries. By 2006 it had more than 170 members worldwide in more than two dozen countries. The first major project of the group was a standardized definition of RLS, which made it easier for physicians to determine who had RLS and who did not. This is critical for research, because you cannot study a condition unless you can decide if someone has it. The RLSF and IRLSSG collaborated and developed a medical advisory board. In 2004, under the direction of Dr. Michael Silber of the Mayo Clinic, the medical advisory board published treatment recommendations.

As it became apparent that RLS was not a rare condition, but instead a common neurological disorder, pharmaceutical companies became interested in the condition. By the early 2000s, several companies had begun trials to see if medications they owned would be effective for RLS. Most of the trials focused on dopamine-enhancing medications. The first to be approved was a levodopa compound (Restex®) in Germany and Switzerland. In 2005 the dopamine agonist ropinirole (Requip®) was approved for use in the U.S. and Europe. The involvement of the pharmaceutical industry definitely benefits people with RLS. Physician and patient education has begun, improving the chances that RLS may be more readily recognized and effectively treated.

It was first reported in 2001 that some families are likely to share the genes that cause RLS. The site of such a gene (on the number 12 chromosome) was first identified by the Canadian geneticist Guy Rouleau, who worked with Jacques Montplaisir, a prominent RLS researcher. Several more genetic sites have since been identified. Although no specific gene has yet been found to cause RLS, at least seven different groups are conducting genetic research.

Another development is the explanation of the connection between iron deficiency and RLS. Researchers from Johns Hopkins and Penn State Universities are working together to understand this connection, assisted by the RLSF "brain bank." A number of people with RLS have been willing to have their brains harvested after death and saved for scientific research. Using this brain tissue, researchers have been able to show that the amount of iron in the brain cells of people with RLS is low; that the brain proteins that keep iron at the right level are not functioning correctly; and that the lack of iron leads to difficulties in developing the contacts between brain cells that are needed for correct brain function.

We now know that RLS is not a degenerative brain disease, such as Parkinson's disease, Alzheimer's disease, or amyotrophic lateral sclerosis (ALS, or Lou Gehrig's disease), but that it probably represents a disturbance in the way the brain works. Future research holds the key to answering the question as to the cause of RLS and treatment.

CHAPTER 2

How Is Restless Legs Syndrome Diagnosed?

ALTHOUGH RLS IS A COMMON CONDITION, many physicians are unable to diagnosis it. (Hopefully, in the future this will no longer be true.) According to a 2001 poll by the National Sleep Foundation, only 3 percent of people with RLS have had the disorder diagnosed by a physician. The REST (RLS Epidemiology Symptoms and Treatment) study, conducted on 23,000 people in four European countries and the U.S., found that 49 percent of the people meeting RLS diagnostic criteria reported they had discussed their symptoms with their physician, but only 7 percent had been diagnosed. This same study found that although 65 percent of those who had significant RLS symptoms two or more times per week had sought help, only 13 percent were diagnosed with RLS. The Night Walker Survey found that, on average, the diagnosis of RLS lagged behind the onset of symptoms by 15–39 years.

> In one study, only 7 percent of the people who discussed their symptoms with their physician were diagnosed with RLS.

There are several reasons for the low diagnostic rate of RLS, including the inability of patients to communicate their symptoms to their physicians. Even when patients do discuss their symptoms with their physicians, it is unlikely that they will receive the correct diagnosis. This clearly represents a huge gap in the knowledge about RLS among medical professionals, resulting in the majority of patients with RLS being left untreated. This can be frustrating and aggravating for those affected by RLS. This gap should improve considerably as more drugs receive U.S. Food and Drug Administration (FDA) approval.

CLINICAL CRITERIA FOR DIAGNOSING RLS

How is the diagnosis of RLS made? This is actually simpler than you may think. Your doctor can diagnose RLS by talking with you about your symptoms. Sleep studies are not necessary for a diagnosis, although they can help. People suspected of having RLS should have a complete physical examination, including blood tests for iron stores, thyroid, liver, and kidney function, diabetes, and a red and white blood cell count.

It is common for physicians to tell patients who have had sleep studies that they have RLS. This is not always correct, because sleep studies may only suggest the diagnosis of RLS. Although sleep studies can detect PLM, not all people with PLM have RLS. Even though more than 80 percent of those with RLS have PLM, these movements may occur as a separate condition, be associated with medical conditions other than RLS, or even be considered normal. In addition, some physicians confuse RLS with PLMD.

There are four essential clinical features of RLS, which are listed briefly in Table 2-1 and discussed in detail below. It is easy to make the diagnosis of RLS once these features are identified. Care must be taken to exclude conditions that mimic RLS, many of which can confuse physicians. In cases where the clinical symptoms are unclear or only three criteria are present, the presence of three other supportive features may be helpful in diagnosing RLS.

Criterion 1

An urge to move the legs, usually accompanied or caused by uncomfortable and unpleasant sensations in the legs. Sometimes the urge to move is present without the uncomfortable sensations, and sometimes the arms of other body parts are involved in addition to the legs.

All people with RLS have an urge to move their legs. It is similar to the urge to scratch an itchy insect bite or move when being tickled.

Table 2-1	Four Essential Diagnostic Criteria for RLS
Criterion 1	An urge to move the legs, usually accompanied or caused by uncomfortable and unpleasant sensations in the legs. Sometimes the urge to move is present without the uncomfortable sensations, and sometimes the arms of other body parts are involved in addition to the legs.
Criterion 2	The urge to move or unpleasant sensations begin or worsen during periods of rest or inactivity, such as lying or sitting.
Criterion 3	The urge to move or unpleasant sensations are partially or totally relieved by movement, such as walking or stretching, at least as long as the activity continues.
Criterion 4	The urge to move or unpleasant sensations are worse in the evening or at night than during the day or only occur in the evening or at night. (When symptoms are severe, the worsening at night may not be noticeable but must have been previously present.)

People with RLS can control this urge somewhat, but it becomes increasingly stronger the longer the legs are not moved. Many people with RLS also have uncomfortable sensations. It is hard for them to describe these leg sensations, and they may use descriptions such as "crawling ants," "wiggling worms," "tight feeling," "an electric current," or "an itchy feeling." Many describe it as an "anxious feeling in my legs," and at first they may think it is just part of a general anxiety problem. As listed in Table 1-1, people with these symptoms and their families often develop pet names for these hard-to-describe symptoms. The sensations are felt deep in the legs, rather than on the surface. They are also usually described as moving inside the leg. As discussed in Chapter 1, only a minority of people describe their uncomfortable sensations as painful.

Sometimes people have a sometimes painful condition called *peripheral neuropathy* (a disease of the nerves in the limbs) associated with their RLS. This can complicate the person's description of his or her RLS symptoms, because the pain from the peripheral neuropathy may seem as if it is part of the RLS disorder. Thus, it can be difficult to diagnose RLS in people who have neuropathy.

Although the name of this disorder includes the word "legs," other body parts can be involved as RLS worsens, including most commonly the arms, but also the trunk, hips, neck, genitals, and rarely, even the face. These parts of the body are almost always affected *after* the legs, and it is rare for people to have RLS symptoms in other body parts without prior involvement of the legs. Although RLS can affect any part of the leg, the feet are often less involved. The symptoms may occur in one leg at a time or both legs together. The pattern of involvement can vary on a daily basis, even in people who tend to have symptoms mostly in one leg.

It is tempting to diagnose RLS in people who have repetitive movements such as foot tapping or rhythmic shaking of a leg. These individuals certainly appear to have "restless legs," because the tapping or other leg movements occur whenever they are sitting. If they are told to stop tapping their foot, they may complain of being uncomfortable because the tapping is calming. This type of foot tapping is quite different from RLS because it is simply a habitual, unconscious behavior.

People who tap their feet can easily stop when they focus on it, resuming only when they become distracted. This is different from people with RLS, who have an almost irresistible urge to move their limbs when sedentary. People with RLS must move or suffer extreme discomfort. In addition, most people with RLS do not use repetitive movements, such as foot tapping, except when confined and unable to get up and walk, because walking is their movement of choice.

Criterion 2

The urge to move or unpleasant sensations begin or worsen during periods of rest or inactivity such as lying or sitting.

People with RLS only develop symptoms when at rest. Usually the symptoms do not occur immediately upon lying or sitting, but take several minutes to develop, depending on the time of day and the severity of the RLS. People with severe RLS may notice the urge to move as soon as they rest. The longer the patient rests, the stronger the urge to move and the more unpleasant the sensations become. The concept of "being at rest" applies to both physical and mental decreased activity. RLS symptoms are more prominent with lying or sitting when there is decreased alertness. Performing mental activities such as reading or playing computer card games can reduce or eliminate symptoms, even when lying or sitting.

RLS symptoms are not related to any specific body position while at rest. Confusion may arise with discomfort or a sensation of "pins and needles" and the urge to get up and move that occurs when lying or sitting with crossed legs for a prolonged period. This is quite different from the RLS discomfort that occurs without any pressure on the legs or specific position.

Criterion 3

The urge to move or unpleasant sensations are partially or totally relieved by movement such as walking or stretching for at least as long as the activity continues.

Most people with RLS will get partial or complete relief from their symptoms almost immediately with movement. The relief will last as long as the patient is moving or engaged in the activity and may return once they are back at rest.

Discomfort from extended lying or sitting cross-legged ("pins and needles") or nighttime leg cramps, which may be confused with RLS, can be distinguished from RLS because they usually do not improve immediately with activity or worsen immediately with the cessation of activity. Walking is the most common activity engaged in for the relief of RLS symptoms, but other actions such as stretching or bending are commonly employed. The type of activity chosen to relieve the symptoms is under voluntary control. Although people can suppress their urge to move for short periods, sooner or later this urge to move becomes so strong that they lose all control and must move.

Some people with RLS may use alternative measures instead of movement. They may rub their legs or take hot or cold—or alternating hot and cold—baths or showers. These coping strategies may provide as much relief as moving and should be considered equal to moving for diagnostic purposes. As RLS worsens, the relief from movement or other measures lessens until these activities no longer provide any relief. Therefore, in severe RLS a history of past relief with movement is acceptable in making the diagnosis.

Criterion 4

The urge to move or unpleasant sensations are worse in the evening or night than during the day, or only occur in the evening or night. When symptoms are severe, the worsening at night may not be noticeable but must have been previously present.

Early in the course of RLS, symptoms may only occur in the late evening. As RLS progresses, symptoms occur earlier in the day until they begin upon awakening. People who have RLS with daytime symptoms find that the symptoms worsen as bedtime approaches. They cannot sit as long, and the symptoms become more intense.

Studies have shown that RLS symptoms peak just after midnight and are at a minimum in the late morning (10:00–11:00 A.M.). These symptoms seem to follow the circadian rhythm, which, in turn, seems to follow body temperature, with RLS symptoms worsening with the fall in body temperature and improving when temperatures are rising. Intense nighttime symptoms often interfere with sleep, causing people to resort to walking at night for relief. It is easy to see why people with RLS have adopted the name "Night Walkers" and why the RLS Foundation uses this name for their newsletter.

Confusion may arise in people with severe RLS, who experience symptoms 24 hours a day without any apparent worsening from morning to nighttime. Like the people with severe RLS discussed in Criterion 3, who have lost their relief with movement, these people will also have a history of worsening in the evening earlier in the course of the condition. This previous history of evening or nighttime worsening is acceptable for diagnosing RLS.

Some people with mild RLS only experience symptoms with prolonged rest and inactivity; for example, when they are on a long airplane trip. If the trip occurs early in the day, they may not yet be aware of their worsening RLS symptoms in the evening. However, if they have extended inactive periods in the evening, they will notice that their RLS symptoms are worse than earlier in the day.

SUPPORTIVE CLINICAL FEATURES

It can be difficult for people to describe their RLS symptoms, making it difficult to determine whether they really have all of the four diagnostic criteria necessary to diagnose the disorder. They may also have other common problems, such as sciatic pain or other nerve-related pains, which may occur in the same area as their RLS, making the diagnosis more confusing. In these cases, the use of the supportive clinical features outlined in Table 2-2 can help confirm the diagnosis. These supportive features are not necessary for diagnosing RLS, but may help when there is doubt about whether a person has RLS.

Family History of RLS

Studies have found that more than 60 percent of people with RLS have a positive family history, with at least one first-degree relative affected with the disorder. It may be difficult to obtain this history, especially from older people, whose parents may already be deceased. However, they may remember one of their parents sleeping poorly, walking a lot at night, complaining about feeling tired during the daytime, or complaining about strange feelings in their legs.

RLS is three to six times more likely to occur in first-degree relatives of people with RLS. Therefore, anyone with a family history of RLS who has leg complaints warrants a closer investigation to determine whether

---

Table 2-2   Supportive Clinical Features

1. **Family History of RLS:** The prevalence of RLS among first-degree relatives of people with RLS is 3-6 times greater than in people without RLS.

2. **Response to Dopamine Drug Therapy:** Nearly all people with RLS show at least an initial positive therapeutic response to a dopamine type (Parkinson's disease) drug used at low doses compared to those used for Parkinson's disease. This initial response is not always maintained.

3. **Periodic Limb Movements:** PLM may occur in sleep or while awake in 85 percent of people with RLS. PLM occur commonly in other disorders and in the elderly, but are much less common in children.

they have RLS. This is especially true for young children with parents who have RLS, because they may not be able to express themselves well enough to describe their symptoms. These complaints may be attributed to "growing pains," when they may actually be treatable RLS symptoms. See Chapter 11 for further discussion on diagnosing RLS in children.

Dopamine Drug Therapy

Many people with RLS will get relief initially from the dopamine-type drugs used to treat Parkinson's disease, including Sinemet®, Parlodel®, Permax®, Mirapex®, and Requip®. These drugs relieve both the unpleasant sensations and the urge to move. The dose necessary to achieve relief is often just a fraction of the dose used to treat people with Parkinson's disease.

In cases where it is not clear whether the patient has RLS, a trial of a dopamine drug may prove helpful in confirming the diagnosis. Relief often occurs at low doses—sometimes as low as half of the smallest strength pills. However, some people may require moderate doses before responding. Even though more than 90 percent of the people with RLS initially improve with dopamine, there will be some who do not respond or need high doses before they obtain relief.

People are often confused because some of the drugs used to treat RLS are the same as those used for Parkinson's disease. However, Parkinson's disease and RLS are quite dissimilar in almost every other way. RLS usually does not show any of the signs of Parkinson's disease and individuals with RLS are not especially likely to get Parkinson's disease. Most important, RLS is not the first sign of Parkinson's disease.

Periodic Limb Movements

As discussed above, PLM occur in more than 85 percent of people with RLS. Thus, when a person's clinical symptoms indicate that he or she may have RLS, obtaining a history of PLM may help confirm the diagnosis. It is incorrect to diagnose RLS in people with PLM who have no RLS symptoms. The PLM merely add supportive evidence when the clinical history of RLS is unclear and the diagnosis is in question. PLM are not specific to RLS and occur more often without RLS. They can occur as a unique entity, with other medical conditions, with various medications, or they may even be considered normal—for example, in the elderly.

When only scant evidence suggests the diagnosis of RLS, the absence of PLM may help eliminate RLS. A sleep study is necessary to assure that the assessment of PLM is accurate. When there are fewer than five PLM per hour, as seen during a sleep study, the diagnosis of RLS becomes unlikely. Performing an expensive sleep study is not recommended just to decide whether an adult has RLS; however, sleep studies do have a role in diagnosing RLS in children.

OTHER CONDITIONS THAT CAN BE CONFUSED WITH RLS

Many other conditions are similar to RLS or PLMD, and they can easily be confused with these disorders. It is usually easy to eliminate RLS if the four diagnostic criteria discussed above are applied to these similar conditions.

Normal People Who Have Repetitive Limb Movements

As discussed previously, normal people who have repetitive limb movements, such as tapping a foot or rhythmically shaking a leg, may appear to have RLS. They clearly have a need to move their limbs and tend to perform these movements whenever they are at rest. People with RLS may use similar leg movements to relieve their RLS symptoms when confined and unable to get up and walk. The difference between people with RLS and normal people who have repetitive limb movements is that the normal people do not have an urge to move their legs, but rather do it out of habit. In addition, they do not have any leg discomfort. If asked to stop their repetitive limb movements, they can easily do so, and may only resume this activity when distracted. People with RLS

> Many other conditions seem similar to RLS or PLMD, and they can be easily confused with these disorders.

must move their legs to overcome the discomfort that has been created by not moving their legs. They may be able to stop the movement for a short period, but by *not* moving their legs they will develop a stronger urge to move them and will also increase their leg discomfort.

Muscular Leg Cramps

Leg cramps are one of the most common medical conditions to be confused with RLS by physicians and patients. Leg cramps may seem similar to RLS in that they cause leg pain and occur predominately at night. The complaints of RLS may be difficult to describe, and physicians often assume that the RLS patient has leg cramps and will treat them with quinine. Some people with RLS may actually use the word "cramp" to describe their leg discomfort because they cannot find a better term to describe it. The treatment for leg cramps does not help RLS at all.

Leg cramps can be distinguished from RLS by the presence of a knotted or tightened muscle in the thigh or calf, with a cramping-type pain in the muscle. Leg cramps generally last for 5–30 minutes and will gradually subside with a change in position—but not necessarily by walking. Leg rubbing may relieve both RLS discomfort and leg cramps, but people with leg cramps will only rub the affected area not the whole leg, as do people with RLS. People with leg cramps may also have a strong urge to move their leg, but when the leg cramping ends, the urge to move and most of the associated discomfort will be gone. People with RLS, however, will continue to have the urge to move and the leg discomfort for many hours, with only temporary relief from walking or rubbing their legs.

Positional Limb Complaints

Pressure on a limb that occurs when sleeping on the limb at night, or sitting with the legs crossed for an extended period of time, is a common phenomenon. Everyone has experienced a leg or arm "falling asleep." The pressure on the limb causes "pins and needles," which creates the urge to move or shake the affected limb. This short-lived urge to move a limb with strange sensations may seem similar to RLS, but unlike RLS, the urge to move and the abnormal sensations will be gone in about 5 minutes. The "pins and needles" will only return if the patient resumes the position that caused the problem in the first place. There is no association with any particular rest position in RLS.

Peripheral Neuropathy

As discussed previously, peripheral neuropathy is a condition in which there is damage to the nerves supplying the legs or arms. This damage can occur from many causes, including physical injury to a nerve, tumors, toxins, autoimmune disorders, nutritional deficiencies, alcoholism, or vascular, metabolic, and endocrine disorders, especially diabetes. Abnormal sensations such as burning, "pins and needles," or actual pain may occur in the affected limb when the sensory nerves are affected. This condition is quite different from RLS in that there is no associated urge to move and the symptoms do not vary with rest and activity. In addition, neuropathy symptoms generally do not get worse in the evening or nighttime, as does RLS.

What complicates the diagnosis of RLS is that a significant minority of people with RLS may have an associated peripheral neuropathy. The abnormal sensations caused by the neuropathy can be easily confused with RLS symptoms because they often occur in the same limbs. It may take excellent detective work to differentiate the symptoms caused by RLS from those of peripheral neuropathy.

Burning Feet Syndrome

This is a common condition characterized by a sensation of burning, heaviness, numbness, and a dull ache in the feet and lower extremities. It often occurs in Asia and during hot weather. This disorder is a type of peripheral neuropathy that mimics some of the features of RLS. The symptoms are often vague and difficult to describe and get worse during the night and better during the day. Despite many of the similarities to RLS, burning feet syndrome can be differentiated from RLS in that there is no associated urge to move and the symptoms do not vary with rest and activity.

Peripheral Vascular Disease

Peripheral vascular disease is caused by blockage of the arteries that supply the arms or legs. At first there is only pain in the legs with walking. However, there will be complaints of leg pain at rest when the condition worsens. Peripheral vascular disease is easily distinguished from RLS in that there is no associated urge to move and, as noted above, walking causes increased pain rather than relieving symptoms.

Fibromyalgia and Chronic Fatigue Syndrome (CFS)

These two conditions are fairly common, have no known causes, and often occur together. People with fibromyalgia have painful muscles, but they are different from people with RLS in that their muscle pain is more generalized, is not associated with an urge to move, and does not vary with rest and activity.

People with fibromyalgia often experience chronic fatigue and have CFS, although CFS can occur without fibromyalgia. The fatigue of people with CFS is similar to that experienced by people with RLS, who are fatigued from sleep deprivation. It is thought that poor sleep quality can lead to fibromyalgia and CFS. It is understandable that many people with RLS can describe their symptoms of fibromyalgia and CFS to their physicians, but not their harder-to-explain RLS symptoms. It may be quite difficult to diagnose RLS in these patients. The symptoms of fibromyalgia and CFS often improve or resolve with the successful treatment of RLS.

Arthritis

Leg discomfort from arthritis shares many features with RLS. Similar to RLS, arthritic pain may get worse in the evening when the person has been active during the day. Many people with RLS are mistakenly treated with anti-inflammatory drugs for leg discomfort. Arthritis can be differentiated from RLS in that it is centered in the joints, rather than more diffusely in the legs. More importantly, arthritis pain gets worse while walking and better with rest, which is the exact opposite of RLS. To complicate matters, RLS has been found to occur more frequently in people with rheumatoid arthritis. These people may feel that their RLS symptoms are related to their arthritis pain, and they do not describe it as a separate problem. It often takes significant further probing to determine that a second problem exists and requires different treatment.

Akathisia

This syndrome consists of a feeling of inner restlessness and the urge to move, which manifests as movements such as rocking while standing or sitting, lifting the feet as if marching on the spot, leg jiggling, and crossing and uncrossing the legs while sitting. Akathisia occurs as a common side effect of the drugs used to treat schizophrenia and other psychoses, antinausea drugs, or when the drugs used to treat Parkinson's disease are withdrawn. The drugs that cause akathisia are generally the ones that block dopamine receptors. They may also worsen RLS.

Unlike RLS, akathisia can occur at any time of the day, usually only when the patient is sitting but not when lying down. The restlessness is generalized and includes feelings of tension, panic, irritability, and impatience. It is not located in or described as discomfort in a limb. People with RLS may describe their symptoms as general restlessness, but they move to relieve the discomfort in their limbs. People with akathisia move to relieve their inner, generalized restlessness.

Painful Legs and Moving Toes Syndrome

This is a rare disorder affecting one or both legs. It manifests as a constant, deep, throbbing ache in the limbs or sometimes burning and involuntary irregular toe movements. The discomfort may be mild or severe, intensifying with activity, and usually ceasing during sleep. This disorder can be easily differentiated from RLS because the discomfort is made worse by walking and does not vary with the time of day.

CHAPTER 3

Who Gets Restless Legs Syndrome and What Causes It?

HOW COMMON IS RLS?

IT IS ESTIMATED THAT APPROXIMATELY 10 percent of the general population has RLS. People who are female, elderly, have a positive family history, or who are of North American and Northern and Western European extraction appear to have a higher chance of developing RLS. Children can have RLS, and hyperactivity among general pediatric patients is associated with symptoms of RLS. Pregnancy, kidney failure, and iron deficiency are among the important secondary causes.

Research studies conducted in Canada in 1994 by Lavigne and colleagues including 2019 people 18 years and older found an RLS rate of 10–15 percent. Fifteen percent of the participants reported restlessness at bedtime, and 10 percent reported unpleasant leg muscle sensations associated with awakening during sleep and an irresistible need to move or walk. A study was published by Phillips and colleagues in 2000 that included 1803 people 18 years and older. The 84 percent response rate in this study yielded an RLS prevalence of 9.4 percent.

RLS prevalence studies conducted in other countries have shown percentage rates ranging from a low of 0.1 percent in Singapore to 10.6 percent in northeastern Germany, indicating that there are some racial or ethnic group differences in the prevalence of RLS. Although more studies are needed to explore these differences, it appears that there may be a lower prevalence of RLS in Asian and Southern European (including Turkey) populations, compared to North American and Northern and Western European populations.

There appears to be a gender imbalance in RLS prevalence, with the disorder occurring up to two times more commonly in women than in men. Two separate studies of Swedish working-age women and men (aged 18–64) found this female preponderance in RLS prevalence with reported prevalence of 11.4 versus 5.8 percent, respectively.

RLS also appears to be related to age. In one study, symptoms five or more nights per month were reported by 3 percent of participants aged 18–29 years; 10 percent of those aged 30–79 years; and 19 percent of those 80 years and older. Another study reported that 53.4 percent of men and 64.8 percent of women (61.1 percent overall) experienced an onset of symptoms at 50 years of age or younger. People whose RLS symptoms start before or at age 45 appear to have more affected relatives than those whose symptoms start later. The age effect for early-onset RLS indicates a slowly progressive disorder. Onset of RLS after age 45 appears to occur less commonly in families and rapidly progresses with age.

Studies have also shown that attention deficit–hyperactivity disorder (ADHD) in children is associated with symptoms of RLS, although the exact prevalence of RLS in children is unknown. (See Chapter 11 for a detailed discussion of RLS in children.)

The Causes of Primary RLS

The causes of both primary and secondary RLS are somewhat mysterious. Other than leg discomfort and sleep torments, individuals with RLS seem to be relatively normal. They often have no other problems with their nervous systems or with any of their other organs. The average person or even an experienced physician would have no idea that someone had RLS when meeting them during the day—unless they began to explain the discomfort they feel at night and their urgent need to keep moving. Sometimes not even close relatives know they are mutually afflicted with this disorder.

The most common form of RLS is known as *primary* RLS, meaning it is *idiopathic*, or of unknown origin. *Secondary* RLS is associated with disorders such as pregnancy, kidney failure, and iron deficiency.

When the authors were doing interviews in a large family, they spoke with two sisters in their 50s. Neither was married and they considered themselves to be best friends. They met frequently and spoke together on the phone at least once a week. Both were severely affected with RLS, but neither knew the other also suffered from the condition because they had never discussed it. RLS is often evident only in the privacy of the bedroom, explaining in part why it has taken so long for it to be recognized as a major medical problem. Physicians cannot *see* the symptoms of RLS, making it difficult to diagnose. Moreover, we now know that the brains of people with RLS appear normal, and it is only when special studies are performed that subtle differences between the brains of people with RLS and others can be observed.

Over the years a number of different causes have been suggested for RLS. Dr. Ekbom believed the disorder was due to poor circulation to the legs. This is a common medical problem that increases in frequency as people age. Although there may be some difference in the way the arteries and veins function in people with RLS, this no longer considered an important cause of the disorder.

Another possible problem for people with RLS is that they may have damage to the nerves in their legs. This is also a common medical problem that becomes even more common as people get older. Studies in recent years have suggested that people with RLS, especially older ones, may have difficulties with some of the nerve fibers going to the legs. There are cases that seem to be influenced by damage to the nerves, for example, the widespread damage seen in neuropathy or with a radiculopathy, also called a "pinched nerve" in the back. However, most people with RLS do not have problems with their nerves.

RLS: A Family Disorder

Many reasons other than inherited genetic makeup can increase the degree to which disorders cluster in families. RLS might be the result of sharing the same environment, eating the same food, breathing the same air, living in the same geographical area, and sharing the same beliefs and attitudes—to some degree. Families share any toxins present in the environment. The amount of light or climate is also shared, as are common medical practices. These factors may be important for RLS, but they have not been explored. Much more effort has been devoted to finding a genetic cause for RLS.

By looking at the DNA of chromosomes, investigators can discover similarities in genes, which could predispose multiple family members to RLS. This means that people with RLS might have similar genetic make-up, whereas people who do not have RLS have different genes. Many of these differences are not important, but some differences can cause significant changes in the makeup of a person or even cause a disease. How does this happen? DNA simply lies in the chromosome, but some is used as a template to make proteins—the real functional elements of every cell. Depending upon the gene, the protein from which it is derived may be normal, vary in function, function badly, be made in too large an amount, or not even be made at all. In this way, how the body works can vary from one person to another because we all have differences in our genes.

Attempts to find a gene by examining DNA have led to at least four links between RLS and genetic makeup. This does not mean that a relevant gene has been found, but rather that individuals who have RLS also share one DNA variant in a specific chromosome. If this sharing is sufficiently strong, and not just something that might occur by chance, this linkage can indicate where on the chromosomes to look for the gene. As of late 2005, regions of chromosomes (numbered 4, 9, 12, and 14) have been found to show such linkage. Researchers are actively looking at these regions for the genes responsible for RLS. Perhaps by the time you read this chapter, one or more genes will have already been found, leading to a treatment for RLS.

RLS and Dopamine

Dopamine is a *neurotransmitter* (brain chemical) that is made in nerve cells and used by those cells to send signals to other nerve cells. It is involved in movement, mood, and alertness. The reason researchers are interested in dopamine with regard to RLS is that the medications that increase dopamine activity in the brain, including levodopa and the dopamine agonists, all seem to benefit RLS. The response of a previously untreated RLS patient to these medications can be quite dramatic. The patient may quickly feel better and may get his or her first night of undisturbed sleep in many years. This response can be so dramatic and so characteristic that the response can be used as a test for the diagnosis of RLS. In addition, drugs that block the dopamine signals in the brain can *cause* RLS.

Attempts to show that dopamine is abnormal in the brains of people with RLS have not brought such clear-cut results. There may be a decreased amount of dopamine in these patients, or there may not. One theory is that dopamine is not decreased, but only shows dramatic swings between day and night in terms of how much is available. Also, autopsies have not found any decrease in the number of dopamine-producing cells in the brain. Indeed, studies of the brains of people who had RLS before death have not shown any large-scale damage to or loss of cells. This is quite different from Parkinson's disease. Although people with Parkinson's also respond to dopamine-enhancing medications, they clearly experience a loss of brain cells, especially those that produce dopamine. Treatment of Parkinson's with dopamine-enhancing medications appears to compensate for the lack of sufficient dopamine, but what these drugs do in RLS is not understood.

In summary, something seems amiss with the dopamine system in the brains of people with RLS, but exactly what this might be is still unknown.

Iron Deficiency in Primary RLS

Iron deficiency has been found in secondary RLS (see next section), but it might also cause primary RLS, and prescribing iron may relieve symptoms. However, researchers believe that body iron might not be the critical issue. In studying the brain, they have found low iron in the fluid that bathes the brain and spinal cord (cerebrospinal fluid, or CSF). Iron has been found to be low in the lower brain when special imaging studies are done with magnetic resonance imaging (MRI) on living people. It has also been found to be low in the brainstem upon autopsy. The brainstems of an RLS patient with low iron and a control who was normal are shown in Figure 3-1. The RLS patient's brain has none of the bright circles and crescents seen in the normal brain. The bright area indicates the presence of iron. Thus, one possible cause for RLS might be the inability of the brain to maintain an adequate iron level. Further studies are needed to determine the role of iron deficiency in primary RLS.

THE CAUSES OF SECONDARY RLS

Secondary RLS is associated with disorders such as pregnancy, kidney failure, and iron deficiency.

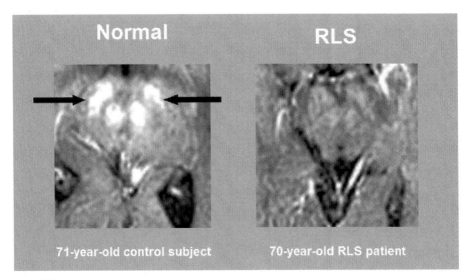

FIGURE 3-1

The white areas show iron in the brain. The arrows point to the substantia nigra; the circular areas are the red nuclei. There is much more iron in the normal brain than in the brain of the RLS patient. (From Allen et al., *Neuroloy* 56:2001.)

Pregnancy

Pregnancy increases the risk of development and exacerbation of RLS in women. A study by Goodman and colleagues in 1988 found that 16 percent of the 500 women interviewed had symptoms of RLS. Their symptoms worsened during the third trimester, but returned to baseline after giving birth in five of these cases.

In a study involving 300 people with RLS, Winkelmann and colleagues found that women who had RLS in their families experienced their first symptom of RLS, or worsening of already present RLS symptoms, significantly more often during pregnancy, compared to women with sporadic forms of RLS. In a separate study involving 642 pregnant women, 26 percent were affected by RLS during pregnancy. Similar to the study by Goodman and colleagues, the symptoms were significant during the third trimester and typically remitted close to the time of delivery.

The cause of the either the development or exacerbation of RLS during pregnancy is unknown. Iron-deficiency anemia is a preventable cause of pregnancy-related RLS, and low iron levels have been observed preconception in women who subsequently developed RLS during pregnancy. There is also a reported association between pregnancy-related RLS and folate deficiency.

Kidney Failure

Overall, studies have reported a 20–70 percent prevalence of RLS in people undergoing kidney dialysis. However, it is difficult to distinguish kidney failure–related RLS from the various sensory and motor abnormalities commonly associated with kidney failure. RLS and PLMD have been shown to be independent predictors of mortality in people with end-stage renal disease. Unfortunately, dialysis does not provide improvement in kidney failure–related RLS, but kidney transplantation may produce significant improvement.

Iron Deficiency

Iron deficiency is found in RLS associated with pregnancy and kidney failure. Individuals with iron-deficiency anemia and those who are frequent blood donors have a high risk for developing RLS. Iron is a key element in the body, and too much or too little can cause problems.

Iron is stored and moved throughout the body in the form of *ferritin* and transported into the cells by *transferrin*. Ferritin is found in two forms: the H-form, which predominates in the brain and is more open for availability of iron and transport, and the L-form, which is used for long-term storage. Ferritin will be low and both transferrin levels and the number of transferrin receptors will be increased when iron is deficient. In 2000 Earley and colleagues demonstrated that the CSF levels of ferritin were low and transferrin levels were high in 16 people with RLS, compared with age-matched healthy control subjects.

MRI studies have also demonstrated decreases in iron content in brain areas such as the substantia nigra and putamen in people with RLS (Figure 3-1).

Other Risk Factors and Secondary Causes

Increased age and positive family history represent risk factors for the development of RLS. In addition, certain rare neurologic conditions, including polyneuropathy, Charcot-Marie-Tooth neuropathy, and spinocerebellar ataxia type 3, as well as medical conditions such as rheumatoid arthritis, represent other risk factors or secondary causes for RLS. The use of nicotine, classes of antidepressants such as tricyclic and selective serotonin reuptake inhibitors (SSRIs), and dopamine antagonists such as metoclopramide may worsen RLS.

Increased age and positive family history represent risk factors for the development of RLS.

The Clinical Course of RLS

The Case of Joe S.

Joe S. is a 62-year-old man who describes "jittery" feelings in his legs to his internist. These feelings are worse at bedtime and when he is at rest, but subside when he moves his legs. Riding in the airplane or car and sitting in a movie theater worsens these feelings. The sensations may prevent him from falling asleep at night, and sometimes he is reluctant to go out at night because he has to "get up and move around." He states that he has had these symptoms since childhood, but that they were mild when he was younger and occurred no more than once a month. The symptoms have gradually but consistently increased in both frequency and severity over time. His symptoms had at least two periods of remission: once when he was in his early 20s, which lasted for almost 2 years, and the other when he was in his late 50s, which lasted for 6 months. Joe S. now has symptoms between 4 and 7 times per week and characterizes them as "severe."

Joe S. describes a fairly typical course for the primary form of RLS, which can begin at any age, although it typically begins in younger individuals. However, RLS does become more common with age. The clinical course of primary RLS varies from person to person, but in most cases it tends to be chronic, and not necessarily progressive. This means that it typically lasts throughout the patient's life, but may not get worse over time. As in the case of Joe S., the patient may experience remissions of his symptoms that last for months or years. These remissions may be associated with relief from stress or result from lifestyle changes. In addition, the causes of secondary RLS may be ameliorated, such as treatment of iron-deficiency anemia–related RLS or pregnancy-related RLS that improves following delivery.

There may be specific visible characteristics in an individual produced by the interaction of the genetic composition of the individual and the environment in primary RLS based on age of symptom onset. A study by Allen and Earley of 26 consecutive patients, 14 of whom had RLS symptoms starting before or at age 45, showed more affected relatives than the 12 people whose symptoms started later. The investigators concluded that early-onset RLS appears to occur commonly in families, slowly progresses with age, and has a limited relation to serum iron status. In contrast, late-onset RLS appears to occur less commonly in families, rapidly progresses with age, and has a strong association to serum iron status.

The Impact of RLS

The REST study of 23,000 primary care patients found 551 people with significant RLS who reported symptoms at least twice weekly and had either some or a high negative impact of symptoms on their quality of life. This study revealed the following:

- 68.6 percent reported taking more than 30 minutes to get to sleep.
- 60.1 percent reported waking three or more times per night.
- 60.8 percent reported that they lacked energy when experiencing RLS symptoms.
- 60.1 percent found it difficult to sit or relax.
- 57.2 percent stated that their daily activities were disturbed.
- 53.9 percent reported a tendency to become "depressed/low."
- 49.7 percent believed the symptoms adversely affected their concentration the next day.

When asked about the overall impact of RLS symptoms on their quality of life, 36.3 percent reported a high negative impact and 63.7 percent reported some negative impact.

Other conditions that were diagnosed in the patients in the REST study included back pain (34.8 percent), depressed mood/depression (26.9 percent), hypertension (26.1 percent), insomnia (26.0 percent), anxiety (23.2 percent), and arthritis (21.8 percent).

The impact of RLS on health-related quality of life was assessed using data from a questionnaire survey and the SF-36 Health Survey obtained from a U.S. sample of 158 people. Relative to the average healthy adult, the unique health-related quality-of-life burden ranged from slightly below normal to dramatically below normal. The unique RLS burden was greater than both type 2 diabetes and osteoarthritis and somewhat similar to that of depression. This means that RLS may have a greater detrimental impact on a patient's quality of life than either adult-onset diabetes or nonrheumatoid arthritis.

CHAPTER 4

Nondrug Therapy and Trigger Avoidance

B EFORE ATTEMPTING TO USE DRUGS for RLS, it is worthwhile to try the nondrug approach, including the avoidance of factors that can trigger symptoms. People with intermittent RLS, who generally have a milder form of the disorder, are the best candidates for nondrug therapy. Even people with severe RLS can benefit from these treatment methods. There are many different strategies that can help avoid or decrease the need for medications.

Some of the techniques described here may be helpful for most people with RLS, but others may only help a few. They are all worth trying because most of these treatments are not harmful. People with RLS can attempt most of these therapies on their own, except those involving medication changes, which should be done only under the supervision of a physician.

ALERTING AND OTHER HELPFUL ACTIVITIES

Mental Activities

RLS occurs with rest and decreased alertness. Thus, RLS occurs during situations that make a person sleepy, including inactivity, repose, and lack of interesting things to see or do. Activities that increase alertness often improve RLS symptoms, because alertness changes the mental state and activates the body's motor system. This can be an important tool for people with RLS, who may find themselves in situations in which they cannot move their legs in order to get relief, such as when sitting on an airplane, in church, or in a business meeting.

Playing video games, doing crossword puzzles or needlework, playing cards, or reading an interesting book are examples of mentally engrossing activities that will usually relieve RLS symptoms. These activities are generally successful for a few hours, as long as a significant level of alertness is maintained. RLS symptoms will return once attention wanes and drowsiness increases. Watching a movie or conducting a normal conversation will probably not improve RLS symptoms—although a heated discussion may be helpful.

Physical Activities

There are many physical activities that can alleviate RLS symptoms. The simplest activity is walking. This will usually relieve symptoms for intermittent RLS, at least temporarily. Unfortunately, there are many situations where walking is not feasible or is inappropriate. With more severe RLS, walking may provide only partial or no relief.

Stretching exercises, including yoga, will often relieve RLS symptoms temporarily. A wide range of stretches can be used, but most apply tension to the calf or thigh muscles. Standing on tip-toe or holding a half-deep knee bend until fatigued are examples of useful exercises. When done before bed these stretches often help people with mild to moderate RLS reduce their symptoms enough so they can fall asleep.

Exercise may be of benefit when performed at a mild-to-moderate level. People with mild RLS may find that a brief walk before bedtime is sufficient to fend off symptoms long enough so they can get to sleep. Higher levels of strenuous exercise tend to exacerbate RLS symptoms, even if done early in the day. Many people with RLS are frustrated when they have to lower their level of physical training in order to avoid worsening their symptoms.

Counterstimulation Activities

A *counterstimulus* is an action that is taken to counter a painful or uncomfortable sensation. An example of this is shaking your hand after hitting a finger accidentally with a hammer. There are several theories on how a counterstimulus decreases painful sensation (sometimes even for hours), but this is not fully understood and is still being studied.

One of the first measures that people with RLS will try when they cannot fall asleep is to rub their legs or get their partner to massage them. This will often provide temporary relief, sometimes long enough to permit sleep. The amount of pressure needed seems to vary considerably, with some people reporting that they need their legs pounded; others prefer milder massage. Some have even purchased electric vibrators/massagers, which may be helpful despite the lack of demonstrated benefit. Leg wraps using Ace bandages, or surgical support hose, are sometimes helpful. Having the feet tickled can bring some people relief for hours.

Baths and showers are frequently used. Most people prefer hot water, but some prefer cold or even alternating hot and cold water. Others have used heating pads or electric blankets. A few people describe using ice packs for several minutes before bed. There are others who must keep their legs free of bedding or other physical contact for relief and in whom massage or other physical contact worsens their RLS symptoms.

Sexual Activities and Orgasm

Many people with RLS find that engaging in sexual activities relieves their RLS symptoms. It is not clear whether the relief is a result of the physical activity itself or the sexual stimulation. Some find that their RLS symptoms return quickly once the sexual activity has ended; many others obtain prolonged relief after having an orgasm. This can be particularly helpful for those with bedtime symptoms.

ABSTINENCE FROM CAFFEINE, NICOTINE, AND ALCOHOL

Abstinence from Caffeine

Caffeine, often called "the world's most popular drug," is the most common of these three drugs that worsen RLS, and the one that most adversely affects people with RLS. Caffeine causes most people with RLS to have increased symptoms, especially if consumed in the evening.

Eliminating caffeine may dramatically improve symptoms in some people with RLS. One physician wrote a medical article in 1978 based on a clinical study of 10 people, in which he concluded that caffeine was the cause of RLS and eliminating it would resolve the disorder. Although no

> Caffeine, especially if consumed in the evening, causes most people with RLS to have increased symptoms.

further reports have confirmed these results, most people with RLS who discontinue caffeine notice significant improvement.

It can be difficult to avoid caffeine entirely, because it is present in significant amounts in many common foods and drugs, both prescription and over the counter. Many people inadvertently consume caffeine and then wonder why their RLS is out of control. People with RLS should familiarize themselves with the caffeine content of various foods and drugs. Charts listing caffeine content can be found on the Internet (see: http://www.cspinet.org/new/cafchart.htm).

Abstinence from Nicotine

Smoking has been associated with aggravation of RLS; however, this effect is not as strong and consistent as that of caffeine. It is still easy to suggest quitting smoking as an RLS treatment because there are many other health benefits from following this advice. Currently, no information is available on whether stopping other forms of nicotine, such as chewing tobacco or snuff, also helps people with RLS.

Abstinence from Alcohol

No studies have been conducted as to the effects of alcohol on RLS, but many people have noted that drinking alcohol increases their RLS symptoms. People with RLS who enjoy having alcoholic beverages will often take extra medication prior to consuming them.

Another concern is that alcohol leads to disturbed sleep, even with a single low dose. This produces increased sleep fragmentation and the number of awakenings in non–alcohol-dependent adults. People with RLS often take hypnotics at bedtime for insomnia, and alcohol is a common choice because of its easy availability. Alcohol intake at bedtime shortens the time needed to fall asleep, but increases wakefulness in the second half of the night. The disturbed sleep and wakefulness in the second half of the night is often further exacerbated by increased RLS symptoms.

AVOIDING MEDICATIONS THAT CAN EXACERBATE SYMPTOMS

Many prescription and over-the-counter medications tend to exacerbate RLS. Many of these medications share a common ability to block dopamine receptors (see Chapter 3 for the role of dopamine in RLS). Physicians are generally not aware of this problem, and it is thus quite common for them to prescribe or recommend drugs that worsen RLS. Patients should learn about these medications and warn their physician.

This section discusses the medications that can worsen RLS and should therefore be avoided. It is common for well-meaning physicians—who may be unaware of the possible triggering relationship between RLS and some medications—to prescribe drugs that worsen RLS. Until medical professionals learn more about RLS, the burden rests with patients to be vigilant and avoid taking drugs that may worsen their symptoms. People with RLS should regularly review their medications with their physicians.

Every patient should obtain a RLS Medical Alert Card, which can be carried in a wallet or purse to serve as a useful reference when traveling, visiting a physician, or seeking help from an emergency room. The Appendix of this book gives information on how to obtain these cards.

"The Value of an RLS Drug Card" by Jill Gunzel, AKA "The RLS Rebel"

RLS Drug Cards are wonderful. I carry and give one to all my doctors. I have had several wonderful moments of sharing it. First, my gynecology–oncologist surgeon studied the card and said, "Hmmm, okay so we aren't going to give you and of the "zine" drugs like Compazine® for nausea; we'll jump right to Zofran®." I told him I had no reason to say any of the drugs *would* cause me an RLS attack, but that I just wanted *everyone* to know they *could*, so that if I started kicking during surgery or recovery, no one would tie me down or write in my charts that I was nuts!

Interestingly enough, as a preparation for my CT scan a couple weeks ago I was told to take Atarax® at night and in the morning. It's known to be almost as bad as Benadryl® for causing RLS. I'd been having RLS for two nights prior to the CAT scan, but after taking Atarax® I slept like a baby. So . . . just because it's on the "no-no" list, doesn't mean it will be bad for you. Still, why not start with the drugs we are pretty sure do not cause problems?

I gave the card to the anesthesiologist right before surgery. He ruled out using Benadryl® and made some notes of his own about the antinausea meds. Six days after surgery, when I had my staples removed, I gave the card to the chemotherapy nurse. First, I told her, "I need to tell you that I have RLS." Her eyes got big and she looked amazed. I thought I'd have to explain it to her, but she blurted out, "Oh my God! I'm glad you mentioned it, because we always give Benadryl® with the pre-chemo drugs and you cannot have that!"

She was very aware of RLS, after having given Benadryl® to a man and having him go bonkers and having to walk the halls with him all night. She also studied the antinausea drugs and noted the color pattern of the fonts on the card. She said, "Most of the usual antinausea drugs are bad for you, too, but you can have Kytril®."

Antihistamines

Antihistamines are the most common drugs that worsen RLS because they are so readily available and frequently used. Some people with RLS may be able to tolerate these drugs, but most will get markedly increased symptoms. They are available as both over-the-counter and prescription drugs and are used frequently to treat the common cold, allergies, and insomnia (Table 4-1). The bottle labels of these drugs need to be reviewed diligently, because they are often used in combination with other drugs.

Table 4-1 Antihistamines That Worsen RLS Symptoms

Generic drug name	Brand name
acrivastine	Semprex-D®
azatadine	Trinalin®, Optimine®
azelastine	Astelin® nasal spray
brompheniramine	Alacol DM® syrup, Bromphen®, Cophene-B®, Diamtapp Cold & Allergy® or DM Cold & Cough®, Nasahist B®, Robitussin Allergy & Cough®
cetirizine	Zyrtec®
chlorpheniramine	Actifed Cold & Sinus®, Advil Allergy Sinus®, Aller-Chlor®, Alka-Seltzer Cold, Cough & Flu® preparations, Chlo-Amine®, Chlorate®, Chlor-Trimeton, Contact Cold & Flu®, Extendyl®, Hycomine®, Gen-Allerate®, Pediacare®, Phenetron®, Robitussin Flu or PM®, Siglet, Sinutab®, Sudafed Sinus & Allergy®, Telachlor®, Teldri®, Theraflu®, Triaminic®, Tussionex PennKinetic, Tylenol Allergy Sinus, Vicks 44M Cough, Cold & Flu®
clemastine	Tavist Allergy®, Tavist-1®
cyproheptadine	Periactin®
dexchlorpheniramine	Polaramine®, Dexchlor®
dimenhydrinate	Calm X®, Dinate®, Dramanate®, Dramamine®, Triptone®
diphenhydramine	AllerMax®, Aller-med® Alka-Seltzer PM®, Banophen®, Bayer Nighttime Relief®, Benadryl®, Compoz®, Diphen Cough®, Diphenhist®, Dormarex®, Excedrin PM®, Genahist®, Goody's PM®, Hyrexin®, Nervine Nighttime Sleep-Aid®, Nytol®, Siladryl®, Simply Sleep®, Sleep-Eze D®, Sominex®, Sudafed Nighttime®, Tavist Nighttime®, Twilite®, Tylenol PM® or Nighttime®, Unisom SleepGels®
doxylamine	Alka-Seltzer Plus Nighttime®, Tylenol Sinus Night Time®, Tylenol Sinus Severe Congestion®, Tylenol Severe Cold & Flu Night Tim®, Unison Sleep, Vicks NyQuil®
hydroxyzine	Atarax®, Hyzine-50®, Vistaril®
phenindamine	Nolahist®
triprolidine	Actifed Cold & Allergy®, Sudafed Sinus Nighttime®

The older antihistamines (also called "first-generation") are the ones that cause the most trouble for people with RLS. The newer second-generation antihistamines (except for cetirizine and acrivastine) do not cross the blood–brain barrier and therefore are much less likely to affect RLS. The safer second-generation drugs (Table 4-2) include the over-the-counter loratadine and the prescription drugs desloratadine and fexofenadine. Nevertheless, some people with RLS will experience an exacerbation of their RLS symptoms with these newer and safer antihistamines.

Table 4-2   Antihistamines That May Not Worsen RLS Symptoms

Generic drug name	Brand name
desloratadine	Clarinex®
fexofenadine	Allegra®
loratadine	Claritin®, Alavert®, Triaminic Allerchews®

Other options for people with RLS who have allergy and sinus problems include steroid nasal sprays, cromolyn nasal spray, montelukast pills, or allergy shots, which can be used to avoid the need for antihistamines (Table 4-3). All of these treatments may be effective for allergy and sinus problems without affecting RLS.

Table 4-3   Alternatives to Antihistamines for Treating Allergy and Sinus Problems

Generic drug name	Brand name
budesonide	Rhinocort Aqua® nasal spray
cromolyn	NasalCrom® nasal spray
flunisolide	Nasalide®, Nasarel® nasal sprays
fluticasone	Flonase® nasal spray
mometasone	Nasonex® nasal spray
montelukast	Singulair® tablets
triamcinolone	Nasacort AQ® nasal spray

People with RLS should be especially wary of over-the-counter sleeping pills because they contain an antihistamine (diphenhydramine or doxylamine) as the active ingredient to promote sleep. People with RLS often seek out these drugs to help them sleep. Unless these pills promote sleep quickly, it is likely there will be a marked worsening of RLS rather than good sleep.

Antinausea Drugs and Antiemetics

These drugs, which are used to reduce nausea and vomiting, are similar in action to antihistamines and block the brain's dopamine receptors (Table 4-4). In fact, some antihistamines (dimenhydrinate) are used as antinausea agents, and many of the drugs in this class have strong antihistamine actions (hydroxyzine). These drugs are also used to treat motion sickness and vestibulitis (inner ear dizziness).

Table 4-4   Antiemetic/Nausea Drugs That Worsen RLS Symptoms

Generic drug name	Brand name
dimenhydrinate	Calm X®, Dinate®, Dramanate®, Dramamine®, Triptone®
hydroxyzine	Atarax®, Hyzine-50®, Vistaril®
meclizine	Antivert®, Bonine®, Dramamine Less Drowsy®
metoclopramide	Reglan®
prochlorperazine	Compazine®
promethazine	Phenergan®
trimethobenzamide	Tigan®

There are alternative drugs for treating nausea and vomiting without affecting RLS (Table 4-5). Domperidone (Motilium®) is not available in the U.S., but it can be purchased in Canada or Mexico. This drug does not cross the blood–brain barrier and therefore does not worsen RLS.

There are three newer antiemetic drugs that are selective 5-HT3 receptor antagonists: granisetron hydrochloride, ondansetron hydrochloride, and dolasetron mesylate. These drugs block the five hydroxytryptamine serotonin receptors but do not bind to the dopamine receptors. People with RLS say these newer drugs work well without exacerbating RLS. Unfortunately, these medications, which are used for preventing nausea and vomiting from chemotherapy, are still expensive.

Table 4-5 Antiemetic/Nausea/Dizziness Drugs That Do Not Worsen
RLS Symptoms

Generic drug name	Brand name
dolasetron mesylate	Anzemet®
domperidone	Motilium® (not available in the U.S.)
granisetron hydrochloride	Kytril®
ondansetron hydrochloride	Zofran®
transdermal scopolamine	Transderm Scop® patches (motion sickness only)

Transdermal scopolamine patches are a good alternative for motion sickness because they do not exacerbate RLS.

Antidepressant Medications

Almost all antidepressant medications can worsen the symptoms of RLS, although this is not understood because they do not affect dopamine

> Almost all antidepressant medications can worsen the symptoms of RLS.

receptors. The most likely hypothesis is that the increase in serotonin produced by many of these drugs is responsible for worsening RLS. This hypothesis helps to explain why the SSRI drugs frequently increase RLS symptoms (Table 4-6).

Table 4-6 Selective Serotonin-Reuptake Inhibitors (SSRIs)

Generic drug name	Brand name
citalopram	Celexa®
escitalopram	Lexapro®
fluoxetine	Prozac®
fluvoxamine	Luvox®
paroxetine	Paxil®
sertraline	Zoloft®

SSRI medications increase the availability of serotonin by blocking the reuptake of serotonin into the part of the nerve that deactivates it. The SNRI (selective serotonin norepinephrine reuptake inhibitor, also called *SSNRI*) drugs, which block both serotonin and norepinephrine reuptake, tend to block enough serotonin reuptake to worsen RLS, as do the SSRI drugs (Table 4-7). Nefazodone may be an exception in the SNRI group, because studies have found that it does not to increase PLMS and therefore may not worsen RLS. However, the use of this drug is now somewhat restricted because of the rare side effect of severe liver damage.

Table 4-7 Selective Serotonin- and Norepinephrine-Reuptake Inhibitors (SNRIs or SSNRIs)

Generic drug name	Brand name
duloxetine	Cymbalta®
nefazodone	Serzone®
venlafaxine	Effexor®

The older tricyclic antidepressant medications (Table 4-8) also have a tendency to worsen RLS. Currently, tricyclics are not used extensively

Table 4-8 Tricyclic Medications and Combinations

Generic drug name	Brand name	Structure
amitriptyline	Elavil®	Tertiary amine
amitriptyline and chlordiazepoxide	Limbitrol®	Tertiary amine
amitriptyline and perphenazine	Triavil®, Etrafon®	Tertiary amine
amoxapine	Ascendin®	Secondary amine/tetracyclic
clomipramine	Anafranil®	Tertiary amine
desipramine	Norpramin®	Secondary amine
doxepin	Sinequan®, Adapin®	Tertiary amine
imipramine	Tofranil®	Tertiary amine
maprotiline	Ludiomil®	Secondary amine/tetracyclic
nortriptyline	Pamelor®, Aventyl®	Secondary amine
protriptyline	Vivactil®	Secondary amine
trimipramine	Surmontil®	Tertiary amine

because they are not as effective as the newer SSRI and SNRI medications, and they have more side effects. These drugs have different effects on RLS symptoms, based on their chemical structure. The tertiary amine tricyclics (amitriptyline, clomipramine, doxepin, imipramine, trimipramine) increase levels of serotonin similar to the SSRI medications, thus tending to worsen RLS. However, the secondary amine tricyclics (desipramine, nortriptyline, protriptyline) significantly increase norepinephrine levels but only produce small increases in serotonin levels.

Although no published studies have yet confirmed this effect, some RLS specialists have found that desipramine does not increase RLS symptoms. The same might be true for the other secondary amines, nortriptyline and protriptyline, which generate only small amounts of serotonin. However, physicians prescribe these drugs much less frequently, and there is not a sufficient amount of experience in using them for people with RLS to draw any such conclusions (thus, nortriptyline and protriptyline are followed by a (?) in Table 4-9).

Table 4-9	Antidepressant Drugs That Do Not Worsen RLS
Generic drug name	Brand name
bupropion	Wellbutrin®
desipramine	Norpramin®
nortriptyline (?)	Pamelor®, Aventyl®
protriptyline (?)	Vivactil®
trazodone	Desyrel®, Trazon®, Trialodinel®

Amoxapine and maprotiline are tetracyclic drugs, but they are often classified as secondary amine tricyclics because they share a similar structure and because they increase norepinephrine levels rather than serotonin levels. These drugs should not aggravate RLS; however, their use has been limited because of the high frequency of significant side effects. Therefore, since it is unlikely that anyone will ever examine the use of these drugs in people with RLS, they have not been included in Table 4-9.

A significant minority of people with RLS do not experience a worsening of symptoms when they take antidepressants; in fact, some may have a lessening of symptoms. This finding is not well understood, but it may be the result of the anxiety-relieving properties of these drugs. Increased anxiety tends to worsen RLS, and thus diminishing anxiety may result in a lessening of symptoms. In addition, many of these medications have significant sedative properties and when taken at bedtime may help promote sleep, causing people with RLS to perceive the improvement in their sleep as a positive effect of these medications.

Mirtazapine (Remeron®) does not fit into any of the classes of antidepressants described above. People with RLS should use this medication with caution, because studies have demonstrated that it tends to worsen symptoms.

The question often arises whether to change the medications of RLS patients who are taking an antidepressant. This needs to be decided on an individual basis. There is no general rule that fits everyone. If the antidepressant drug is truly necessary to treat significant depression, the patient should continue the drug. Increased RLS symptoms resulting from the use of antidepressant medications should be treated in the usual manner.

Some people with RLS may be depressed because of the misery of their unrecognized and untreated RLS symptoms, which the antidepressant treatment may only worsen. After treatment of the RLS symptoms, the depression may improve sufficiently to consider withdrawing the antidepressant medications.

There are some alternative drugs to consider using for people with RLS (Table 4-9). Bupropion enhances dopamine activity, which may improve RLS symptoms. One study has shown that bupropion improved periodic limb movements in depressed people. Trazodone is an older antidepressant that is in a class by itself. Experience with this drug has found that it does not worsen RLS, and it may improve insomnia. One study showed that depressed people had fefwer periodic limb movements when on this medication.

If a person with RLS needs medication for depression, it is probably best to consider bupropion or trazodone. If these drugs are not helpful or well tolerated, another choice might be desipramine. People with RLS who are already on antidepressant medication and doing well should probably stay on their drug regimen. However, if their RLS symptoms remain unmanageable or require a marked increase in RLS medication, a change to a more RLS-friendly medication should be considered, as long as the change does not result in withdrawal symptoms. Alternatively, if a patient is on an SSRI or SNRI medication that is aggravating RLS, the dose can be decreased and combined with an RLS-friendly antidepressant.

Neuroleptic Medications

Neuroleptic drugs treat psychotic conditions such as schizophrenia (see Table 4-10). It is thought that they worsen RLS by blocking the dopamine system. The older neuroleptics are quite similar in action to antinausea drugs. In fact, one of the antinausea drugs, prochlorperazine, is used for both schizophrenia and nausea. These drugs are used to treat fairly serious psychiatric conditions and may need to be continued despite their negative effects on RLS.

One neuroleptic drug, aripiprazole (Abilify®), is a dopamine agonist that may reduce RLS symptoms. There have been many anecdotal reports of people with RLS improving after starting on this drug. If appropriate, it should be considered for people with RLS who need neuroleptic medication.

Iron-Replacement Therapy

As discussed in previous chapters, low levels of iron have been associated with increased severity of RLS. Taking supplemental iron may help diminish symptoms in people with RLS who have decreased iron levels. Not all people with low iron levels will benefit from supplemental iron, and it is often difficult to raise serum iron levels. In addition, RLS symptoms may not necessarily improve when iron levels return to normal.

There are many causes of low iron levels. In women the most common cause is menstrual blood loss, and in men, bleeding from the stomach or bowels. This type of blood loss is usually not obvious because it occurs slowly over many months or years, usually without visible signs.

Table 4-10 Neuroleptic Drugs That Worsen RLS Symptoms

Generic drug name	Brand name
acetophenazine	Tindal®
butaperazine	Repoise®
chlorpromazine	Thorazine®
chlorprothixene	Taractan®
clozapine	Clozaril®
fluphenazine	Permitil®, Prolixin®
haloperidol	Haldol®
lithium	Eskalith®, Lithobid®
loxapine	Loxitane®, Daxolin®
mesoridazine	Serentil®
molindone	Moban®, Lidone®
olanzapine	Zyprexa®
perphenazine	Trilafon®
pimozide	Orap®
piperacetazine	Quide®
prochlorperazine	Compazine®
quetiapine	Seroquel®
risperidone	Risperdal®
thiopropazate	Dartal®
thioridazine	Mellaril®
thiothixene	Navane®
trifluoperazine	Stelazine®
triflupromazine	Vesprin®
ziprasidone	Geodon®

Low serum ferritin or iron levels should trigger a search for a source of blood loss.

Every RLS patient should have his or her serum ferritin level determined by a blood test. This sensitive test for low iron levels measures the body's iron stores. Serum ferritin levels may be falsely increased when people are sick. This test can find low iron levels even when the more commonly performed serum iron level and percentage iron saturation tests are both normal. Most labs will report serum ferritin levels as being normal if they are greater than 10–20 mcg/l, but studies have found that levels of less than 45 mcg/l are associated with an increased severity of RLS. When the serum ferritin level is less than 45 mcg/l, treatment with supplemental iron may improve RLS. Iron can be replaced by the oral, intramuscular, or intravenous routes.

OTHER NONDRUG THERAPIES

Sleep Hygiene

It may seem paradoxical to suggest that people with RLS need to sleep better, because RLS makes it hard to sleep. However, habits can be developed that will make sleep easier for anyone, including those with RLS. The following suggestions can produce a good night's sleep:

1. Sleep as much as needed to feel refreshed and healthy during the day, but no more.
2. A regular bedtime and (even more important) awakening time in the morning strengthens circadian cycling and, with persistence, usually leads to regular times of sleep onset. Bright light in the morning can help stimulate a region in the brain (suprachiasmatic nucleus) that synchronizes the internal sleep–wake cycle with the outside environment.
3. A steady, daily (early in the day, not in the evening) amount of exercise can deepen sleep. Overexertion will not improve sleep because of the resulting muscle soreness and other factors.
4. Occasional loud noises disturb sleep, even in people who are not awakened by noises and cannot remember them in the morning. Sound-attenuated bedrooms, or the use of "white noise," may help those who must sleep in noisy environments.
5. Establish a simple routine that can be followed before bedtime to help you psychologically unwind.
6. Hunger can disturb sleep; a light bedtime snack may be helpful unless you eat something that causes heartburn.
7. Caffeine in the late afternoon and evening disturbs sleep, even in people who do not realize it.

8. Alcohol may help tense people fall asleep more easily, but their sleep will be fragmented and abnormal.

9. The chronic use of tobacco disturbs sleep.

10. Sleeping pills may be helpful, but they can lose their ability to improve sleep if they are taken regularly.

11. People who feel angry and frustrated because they cannot sleep should not try harder to fall asleep; instead, they should turn on a low-level light and do something different. Lying in bed unable to sleep because of stress may produce maladaptive conditioning. The bedroom environment may begin to cause arousal rather than sleep because of its frequent association with frustration and insomnia. The following rules are often recommended to overcome conditioned insomnia:

    a. Go to bed only when sleepy.

    b. Use the bed only for sleeping; do not read, watch television, or eat in bed.

    c. If you are unable to go to sleep after 10–15 minutes, get up and go to another room. Stay up until you are really sleepy, and then return to bed. Choose a relatively boring activity, such as knitting, while you are out of bed; do not start watching an exciting movie on TV. Get up again if sleep still does not come easily. The goal is to associate your bed with falling asleep quickly. Repeat this step as often as necessary throughout the night.

    d. Set the alarm and get up at the same time every morning, regardless of how much you slept during the night. This will help the body acquire a constant sleep–wake rhythm.

    e. Do not nap during the day unless you nap each day at the same time for the same amount of time or you are drowsy and are going to drive or operate heavy machinery.

Complementary and Alternative Medicine (CAM)

CAM therapies are commonly used by people with RLS. Frustrated by the inability of conventional medicine to diagnose and treat their symptoms, people with RLS often turn to complementary and alternative therapies. In addition, people who are taking pharmaceutical drugs may wish to use CAM treatments to reduce or eliminate their need for them.

> Frustrated by the inability of conventional medicine to diagnose and treat their symptoms, people with RLS often turn to complementary and alternative therapies.

Many people consider CAM therapies to be more natural and safer than pharmaceutical drugs; however, some of the remedies listed below may cause side effects and interact with prescription medication.

Complementary medicine is often used in conjunction with conventional medicine; however, alternative medicine can become a substitute for conventional medicine. An example of alternative medicine is treating cancer by using a product such as laetrile, a synthetic chemical related to a substance found naturally in apricot pits, instead of conventional surgery, chemotherapy, and radiation therapy. After numerous people with cancer sought laetrile therapy instead of conventional treatment, the Mayo Clinic performed a study in 1980 showing that treatment with laetrile was the same as giving no treatment at all and that it caused unwanted side effects.

As a result of overwhelming interest and the use of CAM, the National Institutes of Health (NIH) established the National Center for Complementary and Alternative Medicine (NCCAM), with a Web site (nccam.nih.gov) that is informative and offers an excellent resource for research, education, and training. CAM is classified into five categories as follows:

1. *Alternative Medical Systems:* These are separate medical systems built upon theories and practices that differ from conventional medicine. Examples include homeopathic medicine, naturopathic medicine, traditional Chinese medicine, and Ayurveda, an East Indian therapy based on diet and herbal remedies that emphasizes the use of body, mind, and spirit in disease prevention and treatment.

2. *Mind–Body Interventions:* This involves techniques designed to enhance the capacity of the mind to affect bodily function and symptoms. Examples include meditation, prayer, mental healing, and therapies that use creative outlets such as art, music, or dance.

3. *Biologically Based Therapies:* These therapies use substances found in nature, such as herbs, foods, and vitamins. Some of the more popular therapies used by people with RLS are discussed below.

4. *Manipulative and Body-Based Methods:* These methods are based on manipulation and/or movement of one or more parts of the body. Some examples include chiropractic or osteopathic manipulation and massage.

5. *Energy Therapies:* Bio-field therapies, which work on the energy fields that purportedly surround and penetrate the human body, and bio-electromagnetic–based therapies, including those using pulsed fields, magnetic fields, or alternating-current or direct-current fields, make up this category.

There is minimal evidence supporting the use of CAM in RLS and PLMD. Therefore, only anecdotal reports of improvement support the recommendation that a particular therapy is effective for RLS. However, this improvement is just as likely to occur because of the placebo effect as from CAM. Until more studies have been performed confirming the effectiveness and safety of CAM, most physicians will have difficulty recommending these therapies.

Many physicians use CAM in addition to conventional medicine. People who undertake CAM on their own should be cautious. As noted above, the oral CAM medications may interact with prescription drugs or cause other problems. For further information on the safety and use of CAM medications, see the NIH Office of Dietary Supplements (ods.od.nih.gov) or the FDA Center for Food Safety and Applied Nutrition (www.cfsan.fda.gov). Another good source for ongoing information on CAM that is specific to RLS is the RLS Foundation's newsletter, *NightWalkers,* which has a "Complementary Corner" feature (www.rls.org).

Nutritional Considerations

Proper nutrition is often mentioned as beneficial for decreasing RLS symptoms. Despite the fact that there are no studies investigating the effects of diet on RLS or PLMS, this is one of the most frequently attempted interventions by people with RLS.

A common complaint is that ice cream (all flavors) seems to exacerbate RLS. A small percentage of people with RLS believe that decreasing carbohydrates or gluten and wheat (especially white flour) in their diet may be helpful. Many other dietary changes have helped individuals with RLS, but these benefits rarely apply to more than a small minority.

Vitamins and Minerals

There are many anecdotal reports as to the benefits of calcium, magnesium, potassium, zinc, vitamins A, B, C, D, and E, niacin, and folic acid. However, there is no scientific evidence that any of these substances help diminish the symptoms of RLS. A few small studies have suggested that magnesium, vitamin E, vitamin B_{12}, and folic acid may be helpful, but these studies have not been confirmed by larger-scale studies using the best study designs. Thus, it remains uncertain whether supplemental doses of any vitamin or mineral (except iron) can help people with RLS until further studies are conducted.

Herbal Remedies

Herbal remedies are also commonly used by people with RLS, with many anecdotal reports of benefit from kava kava, St. John's wort, butcher's broom, valerian root, horse chestnut, and horse chestnut seed (*Aesculus hippocastum*), Some people have a reported benefit from the amino acid l-tyrosine, pycnogenol (Revenol®), MSM (methylsulfonylmethane), quinine, brewer's yeast, lecithin, coenzyme Q10, and grapeseed extract. None of these remedies have been scientifically studied, and thus they cannot be recommended for use in RLS.

Chiropractic and Acupuncture

Many people with RLS have tried chiropractic or acupuncture therapy for RLS with some benefits, but most people have noted no improvement. There have been no studies using these treatments for RLS, and they cannot be recommended for people with RLS.

Advertised "Cures"

The Internet and popular magazines are full of cures for difficult-to-treat problems, including RLS. Typically these cures will ask you to send money, frequently with a money-back guarantee, in return for receiving an over-the-counter medication or information that is touted to cure RLS. Testimonials from people who have been helped dramatically by the treatments usually accompany these advertisements. People with RLS who are not doing well or who are frustrated with their current medical regimen may be tempted to purchase these remedies. Some of these "cures" do not even list their ingredients or offer evidence supporting how or why their product aids people with RLS. Unfortunately, the manufacturers of these "cures" have never tested their products in a rigorous scientific fashion. The seller's unsubstantiated claims are often the only evidence that the treatment is effective.

The recommendations of people with RLS who have been helped by some of these advertised therapies cannot be relied upon. Unless a treatment has been scientifically tested using a double-blind study—a study where neither the investigators nor the subjects know if the subjects are receiving a placebo (sugar pill) or the real treatment—there is no valid proof of effectiveness.

Double-blind medical studies almost always result in a significant percentage of people in the control group—the group that receives the placebo (sugar pill)—showing improvement. This is called the "placebo effect," and it is actually a common, potent phenomenon seen in all studies of people with RLS. Their claims are real, but that does not mean that the treatment is effective and will work for others? Although some people sustain "placebo-effect" improvements for long periods, most of these improvements will decrease with time.

People with RLS should be wary of all advertised claims for cures or treatments. For those contemplating the purchase of these remedies, the ancient Roman expression, *caveat emptor* (buyer beware), certainly applies.

Chapter 12 discusses other nondrug ways in which people with RLS can help diminish the troubling symptoms of RLS.

CHAPTER 5

Treating Intermittent Restless Legs Syndrome with Medication

INTERMITTENT RLS is defined as RLS that is troublesome enough to require treatment but does not occur frequently enough to necessitate daily therapy. People with intermittent RLS generally have milder symptoms than those with daily RLS and are much easier to treat. Almost all people with intermittent RLS should be able to get relief with the remedies discussed below. More people have intermittent RLS than the other forms of RLS, even though they often do not seek medical attention.

The treatment of intermittent RLS should begin with nondrug therapies (as described in Chapters 4 and 12), which are often quite successful in people with milder symptoms (see Figure 5-1). Although this is the preferred approach, many people will need medications to treat the disorder. Luckily, several different classes of medication are effective for treating RLS.

The spectrum of symptom severity and frequency is quite wide in people with intermittent RLS. Some may have symptoms only once every few weeks; others may be bothered as many as three or more days per week. Clearly, the treatment used for people on the mild side of the spectrum may not suit those on the more severe side. No single drug is best for all people with intermittent RLS. Choosing the right medication from the many available can be difficult. Medications should be selected by matching them to the clinical symptoms and individual needs of each person. Although most people tolerate these drugs fairly well, side effects sometimes limit their use. Some people may need multiple medications because some drugs may be effective or appropriate only in certain situations.

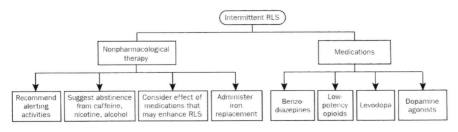

FIGURE 5-1

Algorithm for treatment of intermittent RLS. Adapted from Silber et al., *Mayo Clinic Proceedings*, Vol. 79:2004.

As of June 2006, only one medication, ropinirole (Requip®), had been approved by the FDA for use in moderate to severe primary RLS. All the other drugs that help RLS have FDA approval for other medical conditions, but not yet for RLS. This presents a problem, because many physicians do not feel comfortable prescribing drugs that are not FDA approved, especially when they are not familiar with both the disease and the drugs. The *Physician's Desk Reference* (*PDR*) does not list information on any drug until it is FDA approved, nor does it give any details on how to use drugs approved for other diseases for nonapproved indications such as RLS. The *PDR* is the main drug reference source for most physicians, and thus they cannot easily obtain prescribing information for most of the RLS medications. However, physicians can still learn how to prescribe RLS medications from the many sources listed in the Appendix.

Medications used to treat RLS can be divided into two groups. The first group consists of sedative drugs, which do not improve RLS symptoms but rather promote sleep. Sedatives are appropriate for people with intermittent RLS who develop symptoms when trying to sleep. They can wait until symptoms occur before taking any medication.

RLS medications are most effective when taken before symptoms are anticipated to occur (1-2 hours for dopamine agonists and anticonvulsants and 1/2-1 hour for painkillers).

The second group consists of RLS medications that act directly to reduce RLS symptoms. These medications do not promote sleep, except as an unwanted side effect. These drugs generally have a long lag phase before they start working (30–120 minutes). People with RLS should plan ahead and schedule taking their medications at the appropriate times, because drugs are much more effective at preventing symptoms than relieving them.

BENZODIAZEPINES AND OTHER SEDATIVES

Sedatives are a good choice when RLS symptoms are mild and occur intermittently. The benzodiazepines (Table 5-1) are the most common class of sedative drugs that physicians prescribe to treat anxiety or insomnia. These drugs, which are all related to one of the earliest benzodiazepines, diazepam, also have anticonvulsant and skeletal muscle–relaxing properties. They do not relieve RLS symptoms, but they will help people with RLS fall asleep despite their bothersome symptoms. Once asleep, RLS is no longer a factor unless the patient wakes up. Studies have found that benzodiazepines do not improve the frequency of PLM, but do reduce the arousals from leg jerks and improve sleep quality.

Table 5-1 Benzodiazepines (Hypnotics and Sedatives)

Generic drug name	Brand name	Half-life in hours	Individual dose range (mg)
alprazolam	Xanax®	6-12	.25-1
clonazepam	Klonopin®	30-40	.5-2
clorazepate	Tranxene®	48	7.5-30
chlordiazepoxide	Librium®	7-48	2-25
diazepam	Valium®	24-100	2-10
estazolam	Prosom®	10-24	.5-2
flurazepam	Dalmane®	47-100	15-30
lorazepam	Ativan®	10-20	.5-2
oxazapam	Serax®	8	10-30
quazepam	Doral®	39-73	7.5-30
temazepam	Restoril®	9.5-12.5	7.5-30
triazolam	Halcion®	1.5-5.5	.125-.5

Although people with intermittent RLS may have symptoms from prolonged sitting in the evening, it is usually the bedtime symptoms that are most disruptive and need treatment. These symptoms are generally milder than with daily RLS and may not always prevent sleep. These people need a drug they can take on an "as-needed" basis when their symptoms interfere with falling asleep. Benzodiazepines are ideal for this situation because people can take them when sleep becomes difficult. Additionally, most benzodiazepines work rapidly to promote sleep. Other RLS medications, which relieve RLS symptoms rather than promote sleep, usually take much longer to become effective and should be taken well in advance of the onset of symptoms—

> The short-acting benzodiazepines are very helpful for intermittent bedtime RLS, and they do not cause physical dependence or tolerance when used intermittently.

except for carbidopalevodopa, which may relieve symptoms within 15–30 minutes if taken on an empty stomach. Therefore, these other medications are less suitable for bedtime use for most people with intermittent RLS, who need a fast-acting drug only on those nights when sleep eludes them.

Benzodiazepines are less appropriate for treating daytime RLS symptoms. The risk of sedation, which can impair daytime activities requiring alertness (for example, driving, paperwork, and watching movies), is high. Drugs that do not affect alertness or cause sleepiness are preferred for relieving daytime RLS symptoms.

Benzodiazepines do not relieve the symptoms of most people with RLS; however, they do work in some cases and can be an excellent choice. It is not understood how the benzodiazepines relieve RLS symptoms, but it might be the related to their ability to decrease anxiety. This does not explain how some people experience complete relief of symptoms with benzodiazepines. The benzodiazepines may cause some patients with RLS to fall asleep before their symptoms typically occur.

What is even more puzzling is that studies have also found worsening of RLS with the daytime use of benzodiazepines such as lorazepam.

Table 5-1 lists the benzodiazepines that can be used for treating RLS. Which ones are best can vary based on the properties of the drug and the needs of the individual RLS patient. The first benzodiazepine employed to treat RLS was clonazepam, and, as such, it is the one most often studied clinically. Because of its use in studies and the many medical textbooks recommending it as one of the drugs of choice for RLS, clonazepam has become the most commonly prescribed benzodiazepine for RLS.

Clonazepam promotes sleep fairly quickly, but it has a long half-life, which can be a problem. (The half-life of a drug is the length of time it takes for the body to metabolize a single dose of a drug and remove half of it.) Most drugs are still somewhat effective at one half-life (when the concentration of the drug in the body is at 50 percent), but they will have little impact after two or three half-lives have passed. Clonazepam has a half-life of 30–40 hours, which means it will still be fairly active the next day and thus able to cause daytime sleepiness or decreased alertness. For this reason benzodiazepines with shorter half-lives may be more suitable.

Although there can be considerable variability, drugs with half-lives of about 3 hours tend to work best. Half-lives of all the sedative drugs are listed in Tables 5-1 and 5-2. These values can vary considerably depending on which age group and population was studied to provide the data. Ranges of values are given for many of these drugs to reflect this variability. These values are averages, and a drug's half-life may be different in any individual. People may find that drugs with short half-lives have a long duration of action, and drugs with long half-lives are active for only short periods. Half-life information is useful only as a general guide to drug activity; there are many exceptions.

Of the benzodiazepines, only triazolam has a half-life in the 3-hour range. This drug works well for many people with insomnia and has a low incidence of next-day sleepiness. It may cause *rebound insomnia,* a condition in which insomnia gets worse the night after the medication is taken. Amnesia has also been noted with triazolam, and this can be a troublesome side effect. Because of its short half-life, some people feel that they do not sleep long enough with triazolam. For these people,

71

temazepam may be a better choice because of its longer half-life, which should provide more hours of sleep. Temazepam is not ideal for people who want to fall asleep quickly, because it does not start working for about 45–60 minutes. This may impede its use in intermittent RLS, because people who cannot sleep because of RLS symptoms generally prefer a drug with a faster onset of action.

The benzodiazepines with longer half-lives may be advantageous in people who have anxiety in addition to their insomnia and RLS. Anxiety can be a real problem, because it often makes both insomnia and RLS symptoms worse. The longer-acting benzodiazepines are better for treating anxiety and are used extensively by psychiatrists for this purpose. Daytime drowsiness or decreased mental and physical performance can be a significant problem with the longer-acting benzodiazepines. People are often not aware of the decreased abilities resulting from these drugs and may have difficulties with tasks requiring alertness, such as driving a car. Older people are particularly susceptible to this side effect. Benzodiazepine use has been associated with increased falls and hip fractures in the elderly. Even if they insist that they are having no adverse effects, people who are taking these drugs should be observed closely to make sure they are functioning normally and are not sleepy during the daytime.

Physical dependence and tolerance are also of concern with the regular use of benzodiazepines. Some people can take these drugs daily for many years without any sign of physical dependence or tolerance, while others may have this problem after a relatively short course of therapy. There is no way to predict who will become physically dependant or the duration for which the medications can be used safely. Although physical dependence and tolerance may be a concern when treating daily RLS, this is not a problem when treating intermittent RLS. These drugs do not cause physical dependence or tolerance when taken on an intermittent basis. People who do not take benzodiazepines on a regular basis should not worry about becoming physically dependent on them.

The newer hypnotic drugs offer an alternative to the older benzodiazepines and are not chemically related. They are classified as nonbenzodiazepines hypnotics (Table 5-2) and tend to have fewer side effects

Definitions Approved by the American Academy of Pain Medicine, the American Pain Society, and the American Society of Addiction Medicine, February 2001*

Tolerance: A state of adaptation in which exposure to a drug induces changes that result in a diminution of one or more of the drug's effects over time. For example, after taking codeine 15 mg four times daily for an extended time, you may notice that it no longer results in adequate pain relief and you need 30 mg to get the same effect.

Physical Dependence: A state of adaptation that often includes tolerance and is manifested by a drug class-specific withdrawal syndrome that can be produced by abrupt cessation, rapid dose reduction, decreasing blood level of the drug, and/or administration of an antagonist. For example, in addition to the above-described tolerance to codeine, when stopping the drug you begin to have withdrawal symptoms. These can include increased anxiety, increased heart rate, palpitations, sweating, or even seizures. People who are physically dependent on a drug must continue to take the drug to avoid these withdrawal symptoms.

Psychological Dependence: The result of repeated consumption of a drug which produces psychological but no physical dependence. The psychological dependence produces a desire (not a compulsion) to continue taking drugs for the sense of improved well-being. For example, you may get used to taking a sleeping pill that does not produce physical dependence (such as Lunesta). After a while you may feel that without taking the drug, you will not be able to fall asleep. You have become psychologically dependent on the drug, but stopping the drug does not produce any problems (other than not sleeping) and you do not need higher doses of the drug with time (tolerance). (*This definition is not discussed by the above societies.)

Addiction: Addiction is a primary, chronic, neuro-biologic disease, with genetic, psychosocial, and environmental factors influencing its development and manifestations. It is characterized by behaviors that include one or more of the following: impaired control over drug use, compulsive use, continued use despite harm, and craving. Doctors and others often use the term addiction very loosely in cases of physical dependence and tolerance. However, addiction implies more than just physical dependence and tolerance. For example, the person who is physically dependent and tolerant to codeine may continue to use increasing doses of the medication in order to get relief or prevent withdrawal symptoms. That person does not have an addiction to codeine unless he or she compulsively seeks out more codeine than is necessary to obtain relief from pain or withdrawal symptoms. This behavior of not being able to limit the drug intake to the amount of drug that is sufficient to relieve the symptoms caused by the disease or withdrawal from the drug is what is necessary to diagnose addiction.

than the benzodiazepines and a low potential for physical dependence and tolerance. In addition, they have shorter half-lives and duration of action, which decreases the potential for causing next-day drowsiness. These newer drugs do not yet have a generic equivalent and tend to be more expensive.

Table 5-2   Nonbenzodiazepine Hypnotics

Generic drug name	Brand name	Half-life in hours	Individual dose range (mg)
ramelteon	Rozerem®	1-2.6	8
eszopiclone	Lunesta®	6	1-3
zaleplon	Sonata®	1	10-20
zolpidem	Ambien®	2.5	2.5-10
	Ambien CR®	2.8	6.25-12.5

Zaleplon, with a half-life of only 1 hour, is the shortest acting of the four currently available nonbenzodiazepine drugs. This drug is a good choice for people who have trouble getting to sleep because of their RLS but have no problems with awakening once asleep. People who have both trouble getting to sleep and frequent awakening should consider other medications. Zaleplon can be taken in the middle of the night, and it is relatively safe to take when there are only a few hours left before it is time to get up. This drug rarely causes daytime drowsiness because of its short duration of action.

Zolpidem is one of the most commonly prescribed sleeping pills. With its half-life of 2.5 hours, most people will find that it provides adequate sleep time with little, if any, next-day decreased alertness. However, many people may prefer a longer- or shorter-acting sleeping pill. This is the only nonbenzodiazepine hypnotic drug that has been studied for use in RLS. One small study, which did not use a control group, found it to be effective.

Eszopiclone is the longest-acting of the nonbenzodiazepines. With its half-life of 6 hours, it will usually provide more sleep time than the other drugs in this class, but it has a higher potential of causing next-day drowsiness.

Ramelteon binds to melatonin receptors, so its mechanism of action is different from other sleeping pills. Although its half-life is about 1–2.6 hours, the half-life of one of its metabolites is 2–5 hours. As of June 2006 it is the newest prescription sleeping pill approved by the FDA.

When using benzodiazepine or nonbenzodiazepine drugs, the correct dose is the lowest dose that provides symptom relief. Physicians should initially prescribe the lowest potency tablet (or even half a tablet—except for controlled-release tablets, which should not be split) and increase the dose until they arrive at the lowest dose that resolves the sleep problem. This technique will help ensure that the optimal dose is found and minimize the chances of side effects.

LOW-POTENCY OPIOIDS

Opioids are pain-killing medications that are derived from or chemically related to opium. They are considered narcotics. This class of drugs includes illegal street drugs, such as heroin, and commonly used pain medications, such as codeine (Table 5-3). These drugs are potent for treating pain and RLS, and their benefits have been recognized for many centuries.

> Among the remedies which it has pleased Almighty God to give to man to relieve his sufferings, none is so universal and so efficacious as opium.
>
> THOMAS SYDENHAM (1624-1689)

Narcotics should be used carefully, however, because they are addictive and easily abused. As is the case with benzodiazepines, people with intermittent RLS should not be concerned with these issues, because they will only need to take opioids on an occasional basis.

It is quite common for people with RLS to accidentally discover the benefits of narcotics when given these medications for pain relief, such as after undergoing surgery. Medical studies have examined several of

Table 5-3   Comparison of Narcotic Drug Doses

Generic drug name	Brand name	Usual dose range for RLS	Potency for treating RLS
codeine	Empirin with codeine®, Tylenol with codeine® Codeine Sulfate® (contains no aspirin or acetaminophen)	15-60 mg every 4-6 hours	Low
fentanyl	Duragesic patches®	25-50 mcg/hour patch	High
hydrocodone	Anexsia®, Hycodan®, Lorcet®, Lortab®, Maxidone®, Norco®, Vicodin®, Vicoprofen®, Zydone®	2.5-10 mg every 4-6 hours	Medium
hydromorphone	Dilaudid®	2-8 mg every 4-6 hours	High
levorphanol	Levo-Dromoran®	2-4 mg every 6-8 hours	High
meperidine	Demerol®	50-300 mg every 3-4 hours	Low
methadone	Dolophine®, Methadose®	5-30 mg per day	High
morphine		5-10 mg every 4-6 hours	High
morphine controlled release	MS Contin®	15-30 mg every 12 hours	High
oxycodone	Combunox®, OxyFast®, OxyIR®, Percolone®, Percodan®, Percocet®, Roxicodone®, Tylox®	2.5-10 mg every 4-8 hours	High
oxycodone sustained-release	OxyContin®	10-40 mg every 12 hours	High
pentazocine	Talwin®, Talacen®	50-100 mg every 3-4 hours	Low
propoxyphene	Darvon®, Darvocet®	65-100 mg every 3-4 hours	Low

the opioids and have shown them to be effective for treating RLS. They also modestly decrease the amount of PLM and PLM arousals. It is not clear exactly which of their actions account for the beneficial effects on RLS. They normally stimulate the opioid pain receptors, but blocking these receptors does not decrease their effect on RLS symptoms. In addition, unlike drugs that block dopamine receptors and aggravate RLS, the opioid receptor–blocking drugs do not worsen RLS. It is possible that these drugs work indirectly through the dopamine system, which they are known to act upon.

Many people with RLS prefer the opioids because of their quick onset and reasonable tolerability. They are the fastest acting of all the RLS medications. This can be helpful for people with intermittent RLS when symptoms occur unexpectedly during the daytime and a sedative would be inappropriate. Side effects, including nausea, sedation, dizziness, and constipation, may be less common with the lower-potency opioids used for intermittent RLS. Many physicians are unwilling to prescribe these medications because of their potential for physical dependence and tolerance. See Chapter 15 for information on finding a physician who will prescribe these drugs when appropriate.

As shown in Table 5-3, there are many choices of narcotic medications; the potency of each drug is also listed. The low- or medium-potency medications are best suited for intermittent RLS. The drugs in this lower-potency group are equally effective, although only propoxyphene has been studied for RLS. They all have similar side effects, but some people find after trial and error that they prefer one particular medication.

The correct dose for opioid drugs is the lowest dose that relieves symptoms. If they are available in tablet form, pills can be split to obtain the lowest possible dose. People can take opioids about 30–60 minutes before situations that typically provoke RLS, such as going to a movie or church. Most people do not experience sedation at a lower dose, so they are useful for sedentary activities that require alertness.

Opioids are the most effective drugs to take once RLS symptoms are already present. When used to treat active RLS symptoms, a higher dose is usually necessary than when taken to prevent symptoms. Therefore, people with RLS should always try to anticipate the possibility of RLS symptoms occurring during sedentary activities so they can take their medication in advance. There will be times when people forget to take their RLS medications, and the opioids may be the best choice to relieve symptoms and permit them to continue their activities.

TRAMADOL

Many people cannot take opioids because of allergies or side effects. For these people, the painkiller tramadol (Ultram®, Ultram ER®, or Ultracet®) can be used. Structurally, tramadol is not an opioid, but it exhibits some opioid characteristics. It binds weakly to the μ receptor, one of the three opioid receptors (μ, δ, and κ), but it does so 10-fold less than codeine and 6000-fold less than morphine, which also binds to the μ receptor. Unlike opioids, the pain-killing effects of tramadol are not completely reversed by the opioid antagonist naloxone. Tramadol is as effective as hydrocodone when used to treat pain at a dose of 50–100 mg every 6 hours or 100–300 mg of Ultram ER® once daily. People taking tramadol for RLS should start with one half to one 50 mg tablet and increase to two tablets if necessary.

Although many people with RLS find that tramadol relieves their symptoms as well as hydrocodone, there is great variability in this response. Some obtain more relief with tramadol; others find that it does not help at all. Tramadol tends to have milder and fewer side effects than the opioids—most commonly, nausea, dizziness, drowsiness, tiredness, fatigue, and constipation. Physical dependence is uncommon, but people with a history of physical dependence on opiates should be cautious because they may be susceptible to physical dependence on tramadol.

Tramadol can lower the seizure threshold, and people with epilepsy and those on concomitant seizure threshold–lowering medications—such as tricyclics or SSRI antidepressants, major tranquilizers, bupropion, and opioids—should be cautious when using it. Tramadol is definitely worth considering for use in intermittent RLS, especially when people cannot tolerate opioids.

LEVODOPA

Many studies have found RLS symptoms and PLM to be responsive to dopamine therapy. Dopamine drugs are used to treat Parkinson's disease and prolactin-secreting pituitary tumors. Levodopa was the first drug in this class to be used for RLS. It is a dopamine precursor, which is chemically modified in the body to produce dopamine. When levodopa reaches the brain, the nerve cells convert it into dopamine.

Levodopa normally is combined with another drug, carbidopa, which slows the breakdown of levodopa so that more of it can enter into the brain. This combination medication is sold as carbidopa/levodopa (Sinemet®) and is typically started at ½ to one tablet of 25/100 mg (the first number is the amount of milligrams of carbidopa and the second of levodopa). It is best to take this drug at least 30–60 minutes before RLS symptoms occur so they can be prevented. If quicker onset is needed because symptoms appear unexpectedly, the drug can be taken on an empty stomach to provide relief within 15–30 minutes. Thus, carbidopa/levodopa provides the quickest relief of the dopamine drugs if nausea does not prevent it from being taken on an empty stomach.

Medications that work through the dopamine system can cause worsening of RLS symptoms. This is called *augmentation* (see Chapter 8). Augmentation occurs most often after regular daily use of a medication, sometimes resulting in a severe exacerbation of symptoms. Augmentation may begin within weeks of beginning treatment or only years later. Doses of over 200 mg per day of levodopa (using the carbidopa/levodopa combination) should be avoided, because more than 80 percent of the people with RLS develop augmentation. Concerns about augmentation limit the use of carbidopa/levodopa for daily RLS, but not for intermittent RLS: augmentation should not occur when this drug is used only intermittently at a low dose.

Carbidopa/levodopa is a relatively short-acting drug (3–4 hours). This can create problems for people who wake up after sleeping for 3–4 hours because there is no longer sufficient medication to relieve their symptoms. This is called *rebound* (see Chapter 8), and often an additional dose of medication is needed to treat middle-of-the-night symptoms. In this case, the long-acting, controlled-release preparation of carbidopa/levodopa can be taken. Unfortunately, the controlled-release version does not act quickly and must be combined with immediate-release carbidopa/levodopa. The increased dose exposes the patient to a higher risk of developing augmentation.

Dyskinesia (involuntary movements) is one of the most common and most worrisome adverse reactions reported with long-term treatment of Parkinson's disease with carbidopa/levodopa. Fortunately, this does seem to occur in people with RLS. Nausea is another common problem that can be reduced by taking medication with food.

DOPAMINE AGONISTS

The dopamine agonists, shown in Table 5-4, are drugs that are chemically similar to dopamine and act directly on dopamine receptors. They are not made into dopamine—they substitute for dopamine. These drugs tend to be effective for treating RLS symptoms as well as PLM. They cause fewer and less severe augmentation or rebound symptoms compared to carbidopa/levodopa.

Table 5-4	Dopamine Agonist Drugs			
Generic drug name	**Brand name**	**Half-life in hours**	**Ergot alkaloid derivative**	**Individual dose range (mg)**
Bromocriptine	Parlodel®	3-8	Yes	2.5-10
Cabergoline	Dostinex®	Over 65	Yes	0.25-3
Pergolide	Permax®	7-16	Yes	0.05-1.0
Pramipexole	Mirapex®	8-12	No	0.125-1.5
Ropinirole	Requip®	6	No	0.25-6

When used to treat intermittent RLS, dopamine agonists may be more appropriate for daytime rather than bedtime RLS symptoms. They are not effective for about 1–2 hours and must be taken well before bedtime. If people wait until RLS symptoms occur to take them, they must get out of bed and walk or endure 1–2 hours of symptoms until the drug kicks in. A quicker-acting drug, such as a sedative, immediate-release Sinemet, or painkiller, may be more suitable for people who have bedtime RLS symptoms on an occasional basis.

For daytime situations, such as going to a movie, which will predictably provoke RLS symptoms, a dopamine agonist may be the drug of choice. People can easily take the medication 1–2 hours before the planned activity. Dopamine agonists do not make people sleepy—except for a few, who develop sleepiness as an unwanted side effect.

Based on their chemistry, there are two types of dopamine agonists. This is determined by whether or not they are derived from ergot alka-

> The dopamine agonists, primarily pramipexole and ropinirole, are the preferred medications for moderate to severe daily RLS symptoms.

loids, a chemical produced by a fungus that infects rye and other plants. The ergot alkaloid–derived drugs work well, but they share an uncommon but serious side effect: *fibrosis*, which is the formation of excessive scar tissue in normal organs, including the lining of the lungs, heart, and abdomen, in lung tissue, and on heart valves. People taking these drugs should have an echocardiogram (ultrasound evaluation of the heart) before treatment and at regular intervals while taking this medication to make sure that the drug is not damaging the heart valves. The risks and benefits should be weighed carefully before taking ergot alkaloid–derived drugs for RLS. Most experts only consider using these medications when others are not tolerated or available.

Most of the dopamine agonists share common side effects, including nausea, low blood pressure, dizziness, headache, nasal congestion, hallucinations, and fatigue. Increasing the dose slowly can minimize many of these side effects. Taking the pills with food can reduce nausea. After an initial period of adjustment (1–2 weeks), it is not unusual for many of these adverse effects to decrease in intensity or resolve completely.

Bromocriptine

This ergot alkaloid–derived drug is the first dopamine agonist to be evaluated for treating RLS. It is approved for use in Parkinson's disease and for pituitary tumors that produce high levels of the hormone prolactin. The side effects of bromocriptine are similar to the other dopamine agonists. It should be taken 1–3 hours before bedtime, or before the expected onset of symptoms, such as when going to a movie. Bromocriptine should be started at 2.5–5 mg and increased slowly if necessary, up to a maximum of 15 mg. This drug is not often prescribed for RLS because pergolide and the newer nonergot agonists are available.

Cabergoline

With its long half-life of over 65 hours, this ergot alkaloid–derived drug should not be used to treat intermittent RLS. A single daily dose of this drug may be adequate to treat people with daily RLS who might otherwise need 2–3 doses of the shorter-acting dopamine agonists. Cabergoline can be started at 0.25–0.5 mg in the evening and increased slowly (every 2 weeks) until symptoms are resolved. Studies have demonstrated that it is quite effective at a dose averaging 1.5–2.2 mg per day for people with fairly severe RLS. The side effects of cabergoline are similar to those of other dopamine agonists, with nausea being the most common complaint.

Cabergoline is used more frequently in Europe than in the U.S., where it is prohibitively expensive. In the U.S., drug companies base the price on twice-a-week use for prolactin-producing pituitary tumors. The higher overall doses needed for daily use for RLS are thus too costly, and often insurance companies will only cover use for prolactin-producing pituitary tumors.

Pergolide

This ergot alkaloid–derived drug, which is used to treat Parkinson's disease, has been extensively studied and demonstrated to be effective for treating RLS. It generally relieves RLS symptoms throughout the night because it has a half-life of 7–16 hours. Pergolide should be started at 0.05 mg 1–3 hours before symptoms or bedtime and increased by 0.05 mg every 3–5 days as necessary. Pergolide at its lowest dose of 0.05 mg is equal in potency to the lowest doses of pramipexole (0.125 mg) or ropinirole (0.25 mg). Most people with RLS respond to a daily dose of about 0.25–0.5 mg, but adverse effects (especially nausea) can limit treatment with this drug. The adverse reactions to pergolide are similar to those to the other dopamine agonists, but they are often more intense. People often stop this medication because of side effects. In particular, the association of pergolide and other ergot alkaloid–derivative drugs with valvular disease of the heart has limited its use. People in Europe and Canada can take domperidone (an antinausea medication that does not worsen RLS) to prevent the nausea caused by pergolide.

Pramipexole

Pramipexole was the first of the two non–ergot alkaloid-derived dopamine agonists developed to treat Parkinson's disease and then found effective for RLS. With its long half-life of 8–12 hours, it can control RLS symptoms throughout the night. This medication is a good choice for intermittent and daily RLS. Titration of pramipexole starts at 0.125 mg 1–3 hours before symptoms or bedtime, and then increased by 0.125 mg every 3–5 days as necessary. The side effects of pramipexole are similar to those of the other dopamine agonists, but less severe. Studies have shown that 15–32 percent of those taking it experience augmentation, but symptoms tend to be less severe than with carbidopa/levodopa.

People should be warned that falling asleep during daytime activities (such as when driving a car), at times without any warning, may occur with pramipexole. This usually occurs at doses above 1.5 mg, which is a high dose for most people with RLS. However, increased daytime sleepiness has also been reported with much lower doses. Paradoxically, some people experience insomnia as a side effect of pramipexole.

Pramipexole is now approved for use for RLS in Europe and is being reviewed by the FDA for approval in the United States, which may come within the next year.

Ropinirole

As of this writing, ropinirole is the only drug in the U.S. that is FDA approved for use in RLS. This approval should facilitate the treatment of

RLS by primary care physicians, who are often reluctant to prescribe nonapproved drugs. Ropinirole is not an ergot alkaloid derivative, and there are no concerns about fibrosis.

Despite its somewhat shorter half-life of about 6 hours, most of those who have taken ropinirole at bedtime say it eliminates symptoms for the entire night. This medication is a good choice for intermittent and daily RLS. Ropinirole should be taken at 0.25 mg 1–3 hours before symptoms or bedtime, and increased by 0.25 mg every 3–5 days as necessary. Side effects are similar to those of pramipexole, including concerns with daytime sleepiness. The incidence of augmentation with this drug has not yet been established.

SUMMARY

People with intermittent RLS are a reasonably diverse group. People with symptoms that occur only a few times a month have different needs and concerns than people who have symptoms several times per week. People with intermittent RLS should first attempt nondrug therapies to help them avoid the need for medication or lessen their dosage. Patients and their physicians should choose medications in a logical fashion based on how the actions of the drug fit the needs of the patient. Table 5-5 lists the medications available for the treatment of intermittent RLS.

Table 5-5	Drug Choices for Intermittent RLS
RLS problem	**Drug**
Bedtime RLS	Sedatives, painkillers, or carbidopa/levodopa
Bedtime RLS, 3 or more nights per week	Regular dopamine agonists
Daytime RLS, expected	Dopamine agonists, carbidopa/levodopa, painkillers
Daytime RLS, unexpected	Painkillers or carbidopa/levodopa

People with symptoms that occur only a few times per month usually have two different situations requiring RLS medication. The first is RLS symptoms that occur at bedtime. Symptoms appear only occasionally, and occurrence cannot be predicted. Taking a quick-acting medication to help with falling asleep should be considered if nondrug therapies do not relieve symptoms. Drugs that take 1–3 hours to relieve RLS symptoms, such as the dopamine agonists, are clearly not suitable in this situation.

The best choices for RLS symptoms that occur while trying to fall asleep include carbidopa/levodopa, sedatives, and painkillers. Levodopa compounds work fairly quickly (15 minutes on an empty stomach; 30–60 minutes when taken with food) and are a reasonable choice for many RLS patient when used intermittently. Most sedative and pain-killing drugs work quite quickly, so personal preference should determine which is best for any individual patient. Sedatives and pain-killing drugs are reasonably safe for bedtime use, and physical dependence is not a concern when they are used on an intermittent basis.

Intermittent RLS symptoms can occur after prolonged sitting. People with RLS should be able to predict when these symptoms will occur and plan to take medication in advance to prevent them. The best medications for daytime RLS are the dopamine agonists or carbidopa/levodopa. When taken 1–3 hours before symptoms are anticipated, they should prevent symptoms and also preserve alertness, which is important for activities such as movies, church, and business meetings, but perhaps not for airplane trips. Painkillers are a good alternative. They can prevent RLS symptoms without causing drowsiness when taken 30–60 minutes before extended sitting.

If an unforeseen daytime sedentary situation, such as an emergency business meeting or trip, does occur, or when people forget to take their medication beforehand, the best choices are carbidopa/levodopa or a painkiller. Both of these types of drugs work quickly to relieve symptoms. Most people will not notice a significant decrease in alertness with painkillers.

A different strategy may be necessary for treating bedtime symptoms if intermittent RLS symptoms occur more frequently. When bedtime RLS symptoms start occurring three or more nights per week, the treatment may change to that recommended for daily RLS. People with frequent symptoms can try using dopamine agonists regularly 1–3 hours before bedtime.

Decisions regarding when to begin taking daily preventive medication should be decided in consultation with a physician.

CHAPTER 6

Treating Daily Restless Legs Syndrome with Medication

D AILY RLS IS DEFINED AS RLS that is frequent and troublesome enough to require daily therapy. These people usually have more severe symptoms than those with intermittent RLS. They often require higher doses of medication, often more than once per day. Although treatment is usually more difficult than for intermittent RLS, most people should achieve adequate relief with the therapies outlined in the Daily RLS Algorithm, shown in Figure 6-1.

NONDRUG TREATMENT

People who require daily medication for their RLS symptoms have probably tried the nondrug approach, but their RLS symptoms are usually too severe to respond to these measures. However, the nondrug therapies should be revisited periodically, because there may be older therapies that were overlooked or new ones being developed.

When RLS symptoms occur unexpectedly, using nondrug measures can be invaluable. Medications may not be available or they may be inappropriate, especially if they cause side effects, such as drowsiness when the patient needs to be alert. Even if a medication is available and appropriate, the patient must deal with a lag time of 30 minutes to 3 hours, whereas nondrug therapies sometimes relieve symptoms quickly. People should develop a large "bag of RLS tricks" for these situations (see Chapter 12).

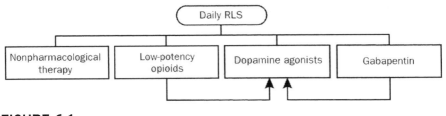

FIGURE 6-1

Algorithm for the treatment of daily RLS. Adapted from Silber et al., *Mayo Clinic Proceedings*, Vol. 79:2004.

DOPAMINE AGONISTS

Dopamine agonists are the drugs of choice for people with daily RLS (see Table 5-4). Numerous studies have consistently demonstrated the effectiveness of dopamine agonists in treating RLS. Almost all people with RLS respond to dopamine agonists—initially at low doses, but as their disorder progresses higher doses may be necessary. Dopamine agonists should be the first class of drugs prescribed for daily RLS unless there is a reason they should not be used.

Although the dopamine drugs used to treat RLS are primarily Parkinson's disease medications, this does not mean that people with

> Pramipexole and ropinirole are the drugs of choice for daily RLS.

RLS will eventually get Parkinson's disease. People with RLS do not develop Parkinson's more frequently than people in the general population. RLS is more common in people with Parkinson's, but they usually develop RLS *after* Parkinson's.

Pramipexole and Ropinirole

The newer nonergot dopamine agonists, pramipexole and ropinirole, are preferred over the older ergot-derived drugs because they have fewer side effects. Many studies have shown that they are effective for treating daily RLS symptoms, even with long-term use. The ergot-derived dopamine agonists should be considered only when pramipexole and ropinirole are not available, too costly, or not tolerated.

As discussed previously, the amount of time that it takes dopamine agonists to become effective (0.5–3 hours) can vary considerably from patient to patient. However, this lag time will remain consistent in any individual person. Once the lag time is established, people with RLS should make an effort to take their medication well in advance of anticipated symptoms. Medications do not work as well if symptoms have already begun. Disruptive RLS symptoms often result when people forget to take their medication on time. For example, people who forget to take their medication before a long car commute may have to stop driving and walk until the drug kicks in. People who forget to take their pills on time should consider wearing a watch with an alarm, or set the alarm on their cell phone, to remind them to take their medication. A stock of medications can be kept in the car, in a briefcase, or another place where they will be available if symptoms arise or if a dose is missed.

Ropinirole and pramipexole usually work well in resolving symptoms. The dose of ropinirole needed is at least twice, if not four times, that of pramipexole. The lowest dose of ropinirole (0.25 mg) is as effective as the lowest dose of pramipexole (0.125 mg), although some experts believe that 0.375 or even 0.5 mg of ropinirole is needed to be as effective as 0.125 mg of pramipexole. In clinical practice, the two drugs generally work comparably at their effective doses, but many people prefer one to the other. It is not understood why this variability exists, but if a patient does not benefit or gets side effects from one of these drugs, it is definitely worth trying the other.

When used to treat daily RLS, these drugs should be taken at their lowest dose (0.125 mg for pramipexole and 0.25 mg for ropinirole) 1–3 hours before bedtime. Elderly people or those who are sensitive to medications may even consider breaking the lowest dose pills in half for their starting dose. If necessary, the dose can be increased every 3–5 days until RLS symptoms are fully resolved. People with daily RLS are likely to have daytime symptoms, and additional doses taken earlier in the day are often necessary. Additional doses can be taken 1–3 hours before symptoms generally occur. The average daily doses needed for pramipexole and ropinirole are about 0.5 mg and 2 mg, respectively; however, the requirements for these drugs can vary considerably; some people may need as little as one half of the lowest dose in the evening; others need large doses three times a day.

Most people find that pramipexole and ropinirole relieve RLS symptoms for about 6–8 hours, although this may vary considerably. Pramipexole may have a longer duration of action because of its longer half-life, but no clinical studies have so far investigated this issue. Therefore, people with RLS symptoms starting in the morning usually need three doses per day, taken at 6- to 8-hour intervals. Although some people may respond to higher doses, most will not benefit from increasing individual doses of pramipexole over 0.75 mg (1.5 mg per day maximum) and ropinirole over 4 mg (6–9 mg per day maximum).

The manufacturers of ropinirole provide a starter pack that supplies 0.25 mg for the first 2 days, 0.5 mg for the next 5 days, followed by 1 mg for the next week. The starter pack insert suggests increasing the dose if necessary (using physician prescribed 0.5 mg tablets) by 0.5 mg on a weekly basis, to a maximum of 4 mg. This titration regimen is based on the drug studies performed to obtain FDA approval, and therefore patients should follow this schedule carefully. This titration plan is reasonable, but it does not allow for as much fine-tuning as the slower method described above, which takes longer to reach a therapeutic dose but might decrease the emergence or severity of side effects.

The side effects of pramipexole and ropinirole are similar to other dopamine agonists (nausea, low blood pressure, dizziness, headache, nasal congestion, hallucinations, and fatigue). Only a small percentage of people who are started on these drugs will have to discontinue them because of unwanted side effects. Nausea can often be averted by taking the medication with food. Higher doses are needed to treat daily RLS, which may increase the incidence of side effects. Daytime sleepiness becomes more likely as the dose is increased, although most people with RLS do not reach dosages that cause this problem (1.5 mg for pramipexole). Overall, despite the potential adverse reactions, most people tolerate these drugs fairly well.

With long-term daily use of pramipexole and ropinirole, augmentation can be a problem. This occurs in more than 15 percent of people on long-term pramipexole (the incidence with ropinirole is not yet known). Augmentation is usually not as severe with carbidopa/levodopa; it can be treated by taking the medication sooner or by adding an extra dose.

Cabergoline

Cabergoline is a long-acting drug that may have a unique role in RLS. It is not used much in the U.S. because it is marketed for twice-weekly use and is too costly to use on a daily basis. In Europe, where this drug is less

> Cabergoline is a reasonable alternative to pramipexole and ropinirole for people with daytime daily RLS.

expensive, it is used much more frequently to treat RLS. This medication needs to be taken only once a day because of its long half-life of 65 hours. This is more convenient for people with severe RLS, who need to take three doses of a dopamine agonist per day. In addition, augmentation seems to occur less with the longer-acting dopamine agonists, which may account for the low occurrence of this problem with cabergoline.

Cabergoline is the newest of the ergot-derived dopamine agonists, and as with the other ergot drugs, there have already been a few reports of valvular heart damage occurring with this drug. People taking cabergoline should have an echocardiogram before treatment and periodically while on therapy. If this drug becomes affordable, it may become a reasonable option for people with daily RLS who have symptoms that begin in the morning.

Even though the majority of people with RLS who are treated with a dopamine agonist get adequate relief, many people benefit only partially or not at all from these drugs. For those people, other drugs must be added or substituted. The two classes of drugs that most experts use in this situation are the painkillers (opioids and tramadol) and anticonvulsants (gabapentin and others). The decision as to which type of drug to use depends upon the patient's symptoms, previous experience with medications, and patient and physician comfort.

LOW-POTENCY OPIOIDS

A significant number of people with daily RLS do not get complete relief with dopamine agonists. Some may not respond fully to high doses; others may be able to tolerate only small doses, which are not adequate to control symptoms completely. Painkillers can be beneficial in these cases. Opioids are effective and safe if prescribed properly. Many people find that they tolerate painkillers better than the other drugs given for RLS. They may experience fewer, if any, side effects from narcotics than from dopamine agonists. As long as physicians follow the prescribing and monitoring guidelines, patients should not fear opioids, but rather take them with confidence.

A few factors may influence the decision to use painkillers. This class of drugs should not be prescribed to people who have had problems with physical dependence or abused opioids in the past. Great care should also be taken with people who have a history of physical dependence or abuse of other drugs, such as alcohol or nonopioid street drugs, including cocaine.

Which painkiller should be added? There is a long list of opioids to choose from (see Table 5-3). These medications should always be started at the lowest possible potency and increased slowly until the minimum effective dose is reached. Opioids can be taken on an as-needed basis for the breakthrough RLS symptoms that the dopamine agonists have not fully controlled. They work quickly and have few side effects. People who get only partial relief from dopamine agonist therapy may benefit from adding a regular dose of a narcotic medication. For people who cannot take a dopamine agonist or do not benefit from them, a narcotic can be substituted and used as the sole RLS medication.

How many times a day should opioids be taken? This varies with the patient's needs and the narcotic that is taken. For the most part, these drugs work somewhat similarly for RLS as they do for pain. The dosing guidelines shown in Table 5-3 can be used as an approximate guide. Most narcotics relieve RLS symptoms for about 3–6 hours and should be taken at those intervals as necessary. Methadone and levorphanol tend to remain effective longer: 6–8 hours. Oxycodone (OxyContin, every 12 hours), morphine (MS Contin, every 12 hours), and the patch containing fentanyl (Duragesic, every 3 days) are available in slow-release formulas, which may be appropriate for people with daily RLS who have symptoms that begin in the morning.

The side effects of opioids include lightheadedness, dizziness, sedation, nausea, and constipation. Sedation may not be a problem with bedtime use, but can limit the use of opioids for daytime RLS symptoms. Constipation is quite common with daily use of opioids, but may be reduced by increasing dietary fiber or taking stool softeners. Nausea can be a difficult side effect to manage, because many antinausea medications tend to worsen RLS.

As discussed in Chapter 5, physical dependence and tolerance should always be considered when taking opioids, which are considered narcotics. These two problems usually occur together. When people become tolerant of a drug, they start needing higher doses of the drug to achieve the same relief the lower doses provided. Eventually, even high doses may not provide relief. Stopping the drug may elicit withdrawal symptoms, which can only be eased by resuming the drug. It is thus easy to understand why many physicians are afraid to prescribe narcotics. This can be a big problem for people with RLS who may require these drugs but whose physicians are reluctant to prescribe them.

There is almost no chance of physical dependence when a person takes opioids intermittently. Although the risk of physical dependence increases when they are taken on a daily basis, it remains low if they are taken only once a day. People taking several daily doses of opioids are at higher risk for developing physical dependence and tolerance. Opioids should be taken at the lowest effective dose, and only when needed to prevent or relieve symptoms. The risk of physical dependence can be decreased by not taking extra doses for other purposes such as mood elevation. Tolerance and physical dependence should be investigated when a person keeps increasing the dose. With proper physician–patient communication and supervision, most people with RLS can take multiple daily narcotic doses without getting addicted.

Often, the biggest problem with using narcotics for RLS is obtaining a prescription. Physicians are reluctant to prescribe them for long-term use, especially for a disorder they do not understand. One solution is for people with RLS to educate their physicians about RLS. Chapter 15 discusses how to find a physician who will prescribe the necessary medication.

TRAMADOL

As discussed in Chapter 5, tramadol has less potential for dependence and abuse than narcotics, but it has medium potency when treating RLS. This less addicting feature may facilitate obtaining a prescription from physicians who are reticent to prescribe narcotics. Tramadol relieves RLS for about 4–6 hours and should be taken accordingly. There is a new form of long-acting tramadol, Ultram ER®, that provides longer relief of about 24 hours per dose and can be taken once daily.

Some people with RLS alternate between taking tramadol and a narcotic, using each drug for several days at a time. Although tramadol is not an opioid, it acts weakly on the same opioid receptor (the μ receptor) as does morphine and the other narcotics used for RLS. It is not clear whether this drug's limited action on the opioid receptors is what decreases its potential for causing physical dependence. Because of the minimal addictive properties of tramadol, it would seem reasonable that alternating it with a narcotic drug would diminish the overall chance of physical dependence. Although this hypothesis has not yet been scientifically investigated, there have been anecdotal reports of people successfully alternating tramadol with narcotic drugs.

GABAPENTIN AND OTHER ANTICONVULSANT MEDICATIONS

Of all the anticonvulsant drugs used to treat epilepsy, gabapentin has been the most studied for treating RLS. Although many studies have shown it to be effective for RLS, its mechanism of action is unknown. It tends to be less potent for RLS than the dopamine agonists or opioids, and is thus more suited for mild to moderate RLS symptoms. However, some people with severe RLS may prefer this drug to the others.

Gabapentin can be started at a dose as low as 100 mg 1–2 hours before bedtime. If needed, the dose can be increased by 100 mg every few days until symptoms are resolved. Most studies indicate that the average daily effective dose is about 1500 mg, but many people benefit from lower doses. The maximum dose generally used for people with RLS is 2700 mg per day. With its half-life of 5-7 hours, this drug is usually effective for 8 or more hours. Two to three doses per day may be necessary for people with early morning RLS.

The high doses of medication that people often need to treat RLS limits the use of gabapentin. The most common and troublesome side effect is sedation, although dizziness also occurs frequently, which limits its use for treating daytime RLS symptoms. When used before bedtime, these sedating side effects may be beneficial for promoting sleep, but because of its long half-life, complaints of morning drug hangover are common.

Despite these potential adverse reactions, many physicians prescribe gabapentin when dopamine agonists are not tolerated or they do not fully resolve RLS symptoms. Physicians often prefer it to painkillers because it is not addictive. The side effect of sleepiness can be of added benefit for people who suffer from insomnia.

> Gabapentin may be effective for RLS, especially for people who experience pain.

Gabapentin has a unique role in treating people with RLS who have pain associated with neuropathy or another unrelated medical condition. Although most people with RLS do not describe their symptoms as painful, a significant minority do have pain. People who develop RLS after age 45 are more likely to have an associated painful neuropathy. Gabapentin may be the drug of choice in these cases.

If a person cannot tolerate gabapentin or it is not effective, the use of other anticonvulsants can be considered (Table 6-1). Most of these drugs have only been evaluated by limited clinical trials or anecdotal case reports. Sleepiness is a shared side effect of anticonvulsant drugs, but the degree of this problem varies considerably with each individual and each drug. It may take some trial and error to find an anticonvulsant that will relieve RLS without causing significant side effects. Because of the lack of clinical experience with other anticonvulsants, the guidelines for using them are not well defined. They should be started at a low dose and gradually increased (usually on a weekly basis) to a maximum, as detailed in Table 6-1. Side effects frequently limit the use of higher doses of all the anticonvulsant drugs.

Table 6-1   Anticonvulsant Drugs

Generic name	Brand name	Individual dose range (mg)
carbamazepine	Carbatrol®, Tegretol®	100-400, up to 3 times per day
gabapentin	Neurontin®	100-900, up to 3 times per day
lamotrigine	Lamictal®	25-250, up to 2 times per day
levetiracetam	Keppra®	250-750, up to 2 times per day
oxcarbazepine	Trileptal®	150-1200, up to 2 times per day
pregabalin	Lyrica®	25-100, up to 3 times per day or 75-150, up to twice daily
tiagabine	Gabitril®	2-10, up to 3 times per day
topiramate	Topamax®	25-200, up to 2 times per day
valproic acid	Depakene®	250-500, up to 2 times per day
zonisamide	Zonegran®	100-600, once daily

BENZODIAZEPINES AND OTHER HYPNOTICS

Although the Daily RLS Algorithm (Figure 6-1) shows the primary drugs used for daily RLS, other drugs may supplement the primary ones. These medications should control RLS symptoms in most people; however, bedtime symptoms sometimes worsen, preventing sleep. For those nights, sedatives can be used on an as-needed basis.

People with RLS are likely to experience chronic insomnia as a result of years of RLS interrupting their sleep. Even after treatment resolves their symptoms, they are sometimes so negatively conditioned to their beds that insomnia persists. There are behavioral techniques for improving chronic insomnia, but people often need sedatives such as benzodiazepines. These medications can be addictive, and the goal should be to use them on an intermittent basis only (see Table 5-1). The newer non-benzodiazepines (see Table 5-2), which have low addictive potential, may be a better choice for people requiring drugs on a daily basis.

OTHER MEDICATIONS

The following medications have been used for RLS in a limited fashion; only a few medical studies have been done on them. Therefore, they cannot be recommended for routine use in RLS, but may be helpful when the more commonly used drugs have failed.

Amantadine

Physicians have used amantadine for many years to treat Parkinson's disease and influenza A. However, the mechanism of its action is not understood. It is not a dopamine agonist, as are the other drugs for Parkinson's disease. One study found that amantadine helped 11 of 21 people with RLS. These patients started the drug at 100 mg and increased it every 3–5 days by 100 mg, to a maximum of 300 mg per day. The side effects found in this study were drowsiness, fatigue, and insomnia. Amantadine may be a reasonable alternative for those who cannot tolerate dopamine-related drugs. More information is necessary before this drug can be recommended for routine use in RLS.

Clonidine

This medication is used mainly for treating high blood pressure. A few studies have found that clonidine relieves RLS. Most of these were case reports; however, one study examined the effect of clonidine on RLS, PLM, and sleep using sleep studies. Researchers found that RLS symptoms were relieved by clonidine, but PLM was not. The average dose of clonidine needed to treat RLS was 0.5 mg per day. One case report described a patient who got relief with clonidine at 0.9 mg per day (in divided doses). Not many physicians treat RLS with clonidine, but this may be a useful drug when other medications are not tolerated or effective. The side effects include dry mouth, drowsiness, dizziness, and constipation.

Selegiline

This drug, which is a monamine oxidase inhibitor, is used to treat Parkinson's disease; it increases the action of dopamine in the body. One study demonstrated an improvement in PLMS with selegiline; however, no studies have demonstrated whether it is effective for RLS. There is extremely little clinical experience with selegiline for treating RLS. A new transdermal patch formulation (Emsam®) has just become available and may be helpful for those who cannot tolerate the oral preparations.

Δ^9-Tetrahydrocannabinol (THC)

THC is the active ingredient in marijuana. No studies have been done with THC to determine its effect on RLS. Many patients have reported that smoking marijuana is effective in eliminating even severe RLS. Many people find that a few puffs of a marijuana cigarette reduces or eliminates their symptoms within minutes. The mechanism of THC's action on RLS is not known, but it has been shown to affect levels of norepinephrine and dopamine. Marijuana is illegal, and people with RLS are advised that they should not use it or risk the legal consequences. Although medical marijuana cards are available in some states, the use of this drug is not sanctioned by the federal government and users are at risk of federal prosecution.

THC is available as a prescription drug, dronabinol (Marinol®). This drug is FDA approved for the treatment of anorexia associated with weight loss in patients with AIDS and the nausea and vomiting associated with cancer chemotherapy in patients who have failed to respond adequately to conventional antinausea treatments.

The effect of taking oral dronabinol capsules is quite different from that of smoking marijuana. After oral administration, dronabinol has an onset of action of approximately 0.5–1 hours, with peak effect at 2–4 hours; the psychoactive effects last for 4–6 hours. Most people do not feel "high" when taking dronabinol because of its slow onset. The effects of smoked marijuana begin within seconds to a few minutes, with higher peak levels than dronabinol.

Anecdotal reports indicate that dronabinol has, at best, a modest effect on RLS. There are no dosing guidelines for using this form of THC for RLS. Dronabinol is available in 2.5, 5, and 10 mg tablets. When prescribed for anorexia, nausea, or vomiting, patients can take it up to two or three times per day with a maximum daily dose of 20 mg.

MEDICATIONS THAT DO *NOT* HELP WITH RLS

The preceding discussion of the treatment of RLS includes all the drugs that studies have demonstrated diminish RLS symptoms. Drugs not mentioned have either not been studied yet or do not help RLS. This includes many commonly used analgesic drugs, such as acetaminophen (Tylenol®), aspirin, and anti-inflammatory medications, such as ibuprofen (Advil®) and naproxen (Aleve®). Although many people with RLS use these over-the-counter pain relievers, they do not relieve RLS symptoms. Several of the painkillers used to treat RLS (propoxyphene, codeine, hydrocodone, oxycodone, and tramadol) are sold with and without the addition of acetaminophen, aspirin, or ibuprofen (Darvocet®, Tylenol with codeine®, Vicodin®, Percodan®, and Ultracet®). The most common forms of these helpful RLS drugs may be the combinations. If possible, it is always better to select the pure form of a medication, which will not contain an additional medication that does not help RLS. The combination formulas expose the user to added risk without possible gain.

Quinine does not diminish the symptoms of RLS, although it is one of the most commonly prescribed. This drug prevents leg cramps, which are frequently confused with RLS. Although there are many anecdotal reports of people showing improvement with quinine, it is likely because of the strong placebo effect typically seen in RLS.

Physicians often prescribe nonsteroidal anti-inflammatory drugs (NSAIDs) for RLS, mistaking the RLS symptoms for arthritis or muscular pain. The NSAIDs include salicylates (aspirin, Bufferin®, and Excedrin®), celecoxib (Celebrex®), diclofenac (Voltaren®, Cataflam®), ibuprofen (Motrin®), indomethacin (Indocin®), meloxicam (Mobic®), naproxen (Naprosyn®), nabumetone (Relafen®), piroxicam (Feldene®), and sulindac (Clinoril®). These medications relieve the pain of arthritis and muscular pain, but they do not benefit people with RLS.

Always check any new RLS prescriptions, and make sure you have been given one of the medications discussed in this book. Also check that any new RLS drug you are prescribed is not on the list of drugs that worsen or do not help RLS. Taking these precautions may avoid a delay in treatment or, even worse, exacerbation of your symptoms.

SUMMARY

People who experience RLS that is severe enough to require daily therapy should first be prescribed a dopamine agonist. Pramipexole and ropinirole are the best choices. These drugs should be started at the lowest possible dose, taken 1–3 hours before symptoms occur and increased if necessary every 3–5 days. People who have daytime symptoms may need extra doses (1–3 hours before symptoms), which can be taken up to three times daily.

If the dopamine agonists fail to relieve symptoms fully, painkillers or anticonvulsants can be tried. The choice of which drug to use depends upon many factors. If patients or their physicians are uncomfortable with opioids, or if there is a history of problems or abuse with these drugs, gabapentin is a good choice. For people with painful RLS symptoms, an associated painful neuropathy, or other pain, gabapentin may be a better option than the opioids. People should always start these drugs at a low dose and increase them only if necessary and as tolerated. If painkillers are not an option and gabapentin is not tolerated or effective, other anticonvulsants can be considered.

For people who do not have problems with painful symptoms or neuropathy, opioids are a reasonable option. Initially, they should try low-potency opioids or tramadol and increase the dose as necessary. Consider the moderate or high-potency opioids for more intense RLS symptoms. Painkillers should always be taken at the lowest dose that relieves symptoms. Most people should be able to tolerate multiple daily low doses of narcotics and still avoid physical dependence and tolerance.

CHAPTER 7

Treating Refractory Restless Legs Syndrome with Medication

THE TERM *REFRACTORY* MEANS resistant to treatment. Refractory RLS occurs when people with daily RLS do not respond well to dopamine agonist therapy. Four main situations result in refractory RLS, as discussed below. Many physicians feel uncomfortable treating refractory RLS and should refer these cases to a specialist. However, by following the algorithm shown in Figure 7-1, many primary care physicians should be able to treat a significant percentage of severe RLS.

INADEQUATE INITIAL RESPONSE DESPITE ADEQUATE DOSES OF MEDICATION

Most people with RLS respond to dopamine agonists early in the course of the disorder; however, with time and the progression of RLS, the dopamine drugs may become less effective or not work at all. People who have severe RLS have symptoms that start earlier in the day. These people often get only limited or no benefit when started on dopamine agonists.

How high should the dose be increased before deciding that the patient has refractory RLS? If there is no improvement in RLS symptoms once the daily dose of pramipexole reaches 1.5 mg, or the dose of ropinirole reaches 6 mg, it becomes less likely that increasing the dose further will help. Although a few people improve after exceeding these doses, most people will need another strategy or medication.

If a person has not responded to one dopamine agonist, he or she may respond to another (see Table 5-4). Both pramipexole and ropini-

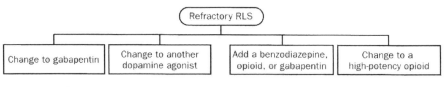

FIGURE 7-1

Algorithm for the treatment of difficult or refractory RLS. Adapted from Silber et al., *Mayo Clinic Procedings*, Vol. 79:2004.

role can be tried, but if they are unsuccessful, other dopamine agonists, such as pergolide or cabergoline, should be considered. However, it is much less likely that these patients will respond to another dopamine agonist. People should discuss the benefits and risks of taking another dopamine drug with their physician. See Table 5-4 for dosing information for cabergoline and pergolide.

Gabapentin or one of the opioids can be tried if the dopamine agonists do not bring relief. The choice often depends on several factors, including the physician's and patient's comfort level with these drugs. The high-potency opioids are more likely to be successful in severe RLS. Physicians who prescribe opioids for refractory RLS can try the low-potency drugs first, but patients often need a higher potency drug. Any of the medium- to high-potency opioids listed in Table 5-3 are suitable for refractory RLS. The ones that are most commonly used are hydrocodone (5–15 mg), methadone (5–10 mg), and oxycodone (5–15 mg). Some RLS specialists prefer methadone for people with severe and refractory RLS. This drug often is more effective than other opioids and has a much lower addictive and abuse potential. It also has a longer half-life that permits longer dose intervals. Tramadol (50–100 mg) or long-acting tramadol (Ultram ER®, 100, 200, or 300 mg) is another choice that may work as well as the opioids for some people with refractory RLS.

To obtain the best results, these drugs should be taken about 30–60 minutes before symptoms occur, up to three times per day if needed. For people who have RLS symptoms 24 hours a day, it may be more convenient to choose one of the sustained-release preparations (fentanyl, sustained-release morphine, or oxycodone), which are taken only twice daily or less.

Physical dependence is a concern at the higher doses needed for people with refractory RLS who have severe symptoms. As discussed in Chapter 6, if these drugs are used properly for people without a history of drug abuse, physical dependence and tolerance and addiction are rare. Psychological and physical dependence can usually be managed if these problems arise. Opioids may be the only drugs that diminish symptoms in refractory RLS. If a physician will not prescribe these drugs because of fear of causing physical dependence or addiction, the patient should ask for a referral to a specialist or find another physician (see Chapter 15).

Anticonvulsants should also be considered for people with refractory RLS. They are also helpful for people with painful RLS symptoms or who have an associated peripheral neuropathy. Any of the drugs listed in Table 6-1 can be used, but gabapentin has been the most studied and prescribed for RLS. These drugs are generally not as potent as opioids for treating severe RLS. This may be a problem for people who do not respond initially to dopamine agonists, because many of them have severe RLS. They usually need high doses of anticonvulsants, which often results in side effects, such as sedation, fatigue, and dizziness, thereby limiting the use of these drugs.

Despite this limitation, anticonvulsants can be helpful for people with mild RLS or when used at low doses in combination with opioids. By adding an antiseizure drug to an opioid, patients can take lower doses of each drug, thereby reducing the potential for adverse reactions and opioid physical dependence.

Sedatives and hypnotics may also benefit people with refractory RLS (see Tables 5-2 and 5-5). RLS symptoms are usually easier to control during the daytime when movement is an option. Bedtime is difficult because the options for movement are limited, and this is also the time when symptoms are peaking. Thus, people may often need extra medication to help them fall asleep. Instead of increasing other medications (opioids and anticonvulsants) on a regular basis, people can take a sedative medication as needed on the nights when RLS symptoms prevent sleep. If necessary, these drugs can be used on a more regular basis, especially when therapy with other drugs is not effective enough or limited by adverse reactions. The choice of sedative or hypnotic will vary depending on the patient's needs. For most, the newer nonbenzodiazepine drugs should be effective and may be safer when used on a daily basis for extended periods (see Table 5-1).

A RESPONSE THAT HAS BECOME INADEQUATE WITH TIME, DESPITE INCREASING DOSAGES

Although many people remain symptom-free for years on low doses of dopamine agonists, it is not uncommon for them to need increased doses with time. Eventually some people may not respond to medication at all. This may happen in a gradual fashion or quite abruptly. It is not always clear why this happens, but there are several possibilities.

Triggers that can worsen RLS suddenly include trauma, such as a car accident or surgery (especially spinal surgery), other medical problems, such as iron-deficiency anemia, and the addition of new medications that are known to worsen RLS symptoms. Tolerance to dopamine agonists can also occur. The patient's history must be investigated for trauma or surgery that may have occurred just before a change in the response to their medications, and all people with RLS should be screened yearly for iron deficiency.

The most common and often the most difficult cause of worsening RLS is when a person takes additional substances or medications that exacerbate their symptoms. It is important that patients and physicians work as a team to find the offending agent. Any drug that exacerbates symptoms should be changed to another that does not cause problems.

If no obvious triggers causing refractory RLS can be found, tolerance or natural progression of the disorder may be the cause. It can be difficult to differentiate between these two problems. Tolerance to dopamine agonists occurs occasionally, but the exact frequency of this problem has not been well defined. This problem may occur at any time during the course of treatment. The mechanism of tolerance is not fully understood, but it is thought that the use of dopamine agonists decreases the sensitivity of the dopamine receptors. Increasing the dose of the dopamine agonist usually overcomes tolerance. However, when tolerance becomes severe, even large doses of medication may not relieve RLS symptoms. When this happens, changing to another dopamine agonist may resolve the problem because there is often no cross-tolerance. For example, if a patient does not respond to increasingly higher doses of pramipexole, changing to ropinirole or pergolide may provide symptom relief. Some people benefit from rotating pramipexole, ropinirole, and pergolide as soon as tolerance occurs (this may vary from several weeks to months).

If changing to a different dopamine agonist does not overcome tolerance, another course of action is necessary. Patients should follow the treatment plan outlined above. The same plan is also appropriate for RLS that has naturally worsened and become unresponsive to dopamine drugs.

INTOLERABLE ADVERSE EFFECTS

Dopamine agonists are fairly well tolerated because people with RLS usually need much lower doses than those with Parkinson's disease. However, people vary greatly in how they tolerate any medication; some have adverse reactions to even the smallest dose of a dopamine agonist. Common side effects, including nausea, low blood pressure, dizziness, headache, nasal congestion, hallucinations, and fatigue, usually occur as the dose is increased. However, some sensitive people have side effects with low doses. Some people may even have unexplained paradoxical reactions to dopamine drugs, with marked worsening of their symptoms when first taking them.

Although all dopamine agonists can cause the same side effects, changing from one to another may eliminate or reduce unwanted consequences. In sensitive individuals, it may take some trial and error to find a dopamine agonist that is not troublesome. Increasing the dose slowly or taking medications with food can help reduce side effects considerably. People who cannot tolerate any of the dopamine agonists should take a different type of medication.

Augmentation That Is Not Controlled with Additional Earlier Doses of a Drug

Augmentation can occur with all dopamine-related drugs (see also Chapter 8). It is so common with levodopa that most RLS specialists will only use this drug at low doses for people with intermittent or mild RLS. The dopamine agonists tend to cause fewer and milder augmentation problems than levodopa. People with augmentation notice that as they increase the dose of levodopa, their symptoms become more intense, start occurring earlier in the day, and may even spread to their arms. When augmentation is mild, taking the drug earlier in the day or taking an additional dose 1-3 hours before the onset of symptoms can often resolve this problem. Augmentation can be severe, requiring larger and earlier doses of medication, until intense RLS symptoms start as soon as the patient wakes up.

> *Augmentation* is a worsening of RLS symptoms that occurs after starting a dopamine-agonist medication to treat RLS. Symptoms can occur earlier in the day, shift to body parts other than the legs, become more intense, or begin after a shorter period of rest.

Severe augmentation invariably causes such distress that people are desperate for relief. Increasing medications further provides little relief and may ultimately intensify symptoms. Stopping the drug will eventually reverse the augmentation, but this may take some time—leaving the patient in great distress. The time it takes for the effects of augmentation to wear off can be quite variable, lasting several days to weeks. Opioids can be used short term to control the intense RLS symptom in these cases.

There are other options for therapy once the effects of augmentation have resolved. Another dopamine agonist may not reproduce augmentation, but it is understandable that many people may be fearful of this choice. Cabergoline (if affordable) may be the best of the dopamine agonists to try if a person has a history of augmentation. Because of its long half-life of over 65 hours, cabergoline probably has the least possibility of causing augmentation, and so far there have been few reports of this problem. Treatment with either a narcotic or an anticonvulsant should be started if dopamine agonists are no longer an option after augmentation has occurred. (See Chapter 8 for further discussion of augmentation.)

COMBINATION THERAPY

The advantage of combination therapy is that people can often take lower, better-tolerated doses of medications and get relief that is not provided by one medication alone. For some people, medications may partially improve RLS symptoms at lower doses, but higher doses may not be tolerated or provide adequate relief. Instead of stopping a medication that is only partially effective at a low dose, it may be appropriate to add additional medications. These additional drugs can be added at lower dosages, especially in people who are sensitive to side effects, or in higher doses for those who tolerate them and have severe, refractory RLS.

In addition, individual symptoms can be more specifically targeted with combination therapy. Painful neuropathy complaints may be better treated with gabapentin or other anticonvulsants. Insomnia should respond well to one of the hypnotic drugs, or even an RLS drug such as gabapentin, which can cause sedation. Daytime symptoms may be more appropriately treated with drugs that do not cause sedation. However, trial and error is often required to find the correct combination of drugs, because the therapeutic benefits and side effects of these medications vary considerably from one person to the next.

Usually, a dopamine agonist (unless not tolerated or completely ineffective) is at the core of combination therapy. However, combinations without dopaminergic medication are also sometimes helpful. The dopamine agonist should be taken at the highest dose that can be comfortably tolerated. When this dose is not adequately effective, another medication can be added. Painkillers can be taken at their lowest effective dose, often up to three to four times per day as needed. Most people do not get sleepy from taking painkillers, so they are usually a good choice for daytime symptoms, especially unexpected symptoms, because they work quickly. Gabapentin or another anticonvulsant can also be added to the combination and taken two to three times per day. Sedation often limits the daytime use of higher doses of these drugs; thus, lower doses should be prescribed, or higher doses should be taken 1–3 hours before bedtime, which may be helpful for people with insomnia. For those nights when a person has increased RLS symptoms that prevent sleep, a hypnotic (benzodiazepine or nonbenzodiazepine) may be helpful. Treatment that provides quick relief for unexpected RLS symptoms should also be prescribed. Levodopa (Sinemet®), painkillers, or hypnotics for bedtime symptoms may be effective.

People with RLS who have problems with anxiety and depression may find that their RLS symptoms improve if they are treated with a dopamine-active antidepressant drug, such as bupropion (Wellbutrin®).

Remember, we all respond differently to medications, and physicians cannot always predict which medication or combination of medications will suit any given individual. Using the above guidelines should facilitate arriving at the optimal combination therapy, but it may still take considerable trial and error to get there.

Summary

There is no set formula for refractory RLS therapy. Each patient should have an individualized treatment plan based on his or her needs and drug tolerance. Physicians should use the algorithm shown in Figure 7-1 as a guide for selecting the medication to prescribe.

Dopamine agonists are the drugs of choice for refractory RLS. Physicians should select one based on effectiveness, safety, side effect profile, availability, cost, and their comfort level with the drug. Dosages can be increased slowly until symptoms are resolved. When people cannot tolerate their medications, or the drugs become less effective, they should seek alternative therapy. If one dopamine agonist causes side effects or does not relieve symptoms, physicians should consider prescribing another drug instead. Once two or more dopamine drugs have been unsuccessful, another course of therapy should be considered, such as an opioid or anticonvulsant. The choice of which drug to use depends upon the patient's history, especially if there has been previous physical dependence, severity of the RLS, and the comfort level of both the patient and the physician with these drugs.

Narcotics may be a good choice for people with severe RLS. Physicians should consider lower-potency opioids first, but if they are not helpful, more potent ones can be prescribed. Some RLS specialists prefer the use of methadone. Opioids should always be taken in the lowest dose that relieves symptoms. Physical dependence is a concern, but this can be minimized with proper care and monitoring. Many people become psychologically dependent on opioids because they provide dramatic symptom relief. These concerns should not be an impediment that prevents people from receiving the help they need.

People with less intense RLS symptoms may respond well to anticonvulsants. Physicians should always consider these drugs for patients with painful RLS symptoms or those who have an associated painful peripheral neuropathy. Additionally, when people do not tolerate narcotics or should not take them because of previous physical dependence problems, anticonvulsants should be considered. Side effects can be limited by starting at a low dose and increasing slowly.

There is great variability in how people respond to medications. What works for one patient may cause problems in another. Flexibility in treatment is important for success. Frequently, drugs must be used in combination to achieve control of symptoms. If one drug is partially effective, adding another drug may relieve RLS symptoms in addition to reducing the emergence of side effects. Many people do well with low doses of a dopamine agonist combined with either opioids or anticonvulsants. Some people do better when taking both an opioid and anticonvulsant with a dopamine agonist. In addition, people should consider sedatives or hypnotics when their symptoms prevent them from sleeping.

CHAPTER 8

Augmentation, Rebound, and Tolerance

T HESE TERMS APPLY TO PROBLEMS that occur with dopamine therapy for RLS, and they tend to be confused with one another. Although they share many similarities, they have distinct characteristics that allow them to be readily differentiated from one another. This chapter discusses how to recognize and deal with these troublesome side effects of dopamine treatment.

AUGMENTATION

Augmentation tends to cause the most common and severe problems in RLS treatment. *Augmentation* is defined as a worsening of RLS symptoms that is related to a therapy given to treat these symptoms. So far, almost all augmentation is caused by dopaminergic drugs; the only other drug reported to cause augmentation in a small case series was tramadol. The most characteristic worsening with augmentation is the occurrence of symptoms earlier in the day than before the onset of treatment. Therefore, someone who used to have symptoms only at bedtime may find that after taking a drug that acts on the dopamine system, the symptoms start occurring several hours before bedtime. The different features of augmentation are described in Table 8-1.

Previous determinations of augmentation have relied upon a physician's judgment to decide whether it was present, because there were no standards to guide them. In 2005, however, a scale was tested in Europe: the Augmentation Severity Rating Scale (ASRS). This scale can be used to measure the degree of augmentation.

Augmentation occurs most frequently with levodopa. In clinical use, levodopa is almost always taken as a combination medication with

Table 8-1   Key Features for Augmentation of RLS

1. Earlier onset of symptoms
2. Increased severity of symptoms
3. Reduced time before symptoms begin when resting
4. Spread of symptoms to previously uninvolved body parts (for example, someone who had RLS only in the legs begins to develop symptoms in the arms)
5. Reduced effectiveness of medications, including longer time before medication begins to work and less ability to decrease symptoms
6. Abrupt and often dramatic increase in symptoms immediately after the drug is withdrawn, followed by a return to less severe symptoms days to weeks later

another drug that reduces its side effects by decreasing the amount of levodopa needed for a therapeutic effect (carbidopa in the U.S. and benserazide in Europe). The most familiar form of levodopa is the brand name drug Sinemet®. The combined drug is usually designated by two numbers, such as 25/100. The first refers to the second drug, carbidopa in the U.S., and the second figure to levodopa; thus, 25/100 pills have 100 milligrams of levodopa.

Studies show that between 27 and 82 percent of the people taking this drug develop augmentation. Levodopa readily causes augmentation when the daily dose exceeds 200 mg (two 25/100 tablets of Sinemet®). Augmentation from levodopa causes much more intense symptoms, with a rapid shift of symptoms to earlier in the day, compared to augmentation caused by dopamine agonists. Augmentation from levodopa usually produces much more distress than that from the dopamine agonists. RLS symptoms can occur around the clock, and further increases in the dose of levodopa provide only temporary relief. People commonly describe severe augmentation as a "living hell." It is thought that this increase in all aspects of augmentation with levodopa may be the result of its short half-life. Because of the severity of the augmentation from levodopa, people should use this drug with great caution, especially with daily doses over 200 mg. Of course, if a patient is happy with levodopa treatment, there is no reason to stop using it.

Rates of augmentation are much lower with the dopamine agonists compared to levodopa. Augmentation has been reported to occur with pergolide at 0–27 percent, pramipexole at 0–39 percent, ropinirole at 0–10 percent, and cabergoline at 0–9 percent. These augmentation rates have wide ranges of values because previous studies used different criteria for diagnosing this problem. It is likely that the frequency of augmentation is closer to the higher level and not the lower. Future research papers on augmentation should be more standardized, using the International Restless Legs Study Group criteria and the ASRS. Until then, it is difficult to compare one dopamine agonist with another. However, it is generally agreed that none of them cause as much augmentation as levodopa. Since it is thought that dopamine drugs with longer half-lives are less likely to produce augmentation, cabergoline, with its 65-hour half-life, may be the least likely to cause this difficulty. One aspect of longer half-lives is that drug levels in the blood do not rise and fall as rapidly, but remain fairly steady. Another way to achieve even levels is to use continuous-release medication. Rotigotine is one such drug currently under study. This non–ergot dopamine agonist comes as a patch that is worn around the clock, continuously releasing the medication for 24 hours.

Augmentation frequently occurs within 6 months after the beginning of treatment or an increase in dosage; however, it can occur at any time during the course of therapy, including within the first week. Augmentation tends to occur more rapidly in combinations containing levodopa, usually within the first 2 months of therapy. One of the few studies examining the long-term use of a dopamine agonist in RLS (Pramipexole in the Management of Restless Legs Syndrome: An Extended Study; 2003) found that the augmentation rate with pramipexole was 20 percent in the first year, which dropped to 10 percent in the second year, and no new cases developed after 2½ years. Later worsening of symptoms may be the result of tolerance to the medication—a simple loss of effectiveness without worsening of the patient's RLS—or to progression of the RLS. One key difference between tolerance and augmentation is that tolerance does not change the timing of symptoms, and the symptoms should not become more severe than before treatment began. Although augmentation often results in an increase in the intensity of the RLS symptoms (Table 8-1, Feature 2), this is not always the case. For some people augmentation may include other key features, rather than an increase in RLS symptom intensity.

Before diagnosing augmentation, physicians should exclude other conditions or situations that may aggravate RLS, because these can easily mimic augmentation. They must also rule out natural worsening of RLS, which tends to occur with time in many people. This can be difficult to differentiate from augmentation, because when RLS worsens naturally, people require higher doses of the dopamine drugs. With augmentation, the intensity of symptoms should diminish when people decrease the dose of their medication. However, many people go through an acute withdrawal period that can last several days or longer after discontinuing their dopamine medications before achieving a decrease in the intensity of their RLS symptoms. Their symptoms usually become even more severe during the withdrawal period.

Other factors that temporarily worsen RLS must also be ruled out. A search for medications that worsen RLS should be done, as this is a common occurrence that can imitate augmentation. Caffeine, alcohol, and tobacco should also be ruled out as possible causes of worsening RLS before assuming that augmentation is to blame. Iron levels should also be tested.

Last night was one of those horrible nights. Nights this severe are becoming more frequent and it scares me. I keep feeling that there has got to be something out there that I can take each night and simply fall asleep like normal people do. I really don't feel like I can go on much further without some good quality of sleep.

49-year-old woman, Dayton, Ohio

What can a physician do when a patient develops augmentation? This depends upon the severity of symptoms and the impact they have on the person's life. When symptoms are severe and disruptive, people should stop taking the potentially problematic dopamine drug. This will resolve the augmentation problem, but it may take several days or even longer. During this interval, they may need additional therapy to control the severe RLS symptoms that result from withdrawal. Medium- to high-potency opioids (see Table 5-3) are usually the best choice for this situation. These drugs work quickly and effectively to control the increased RLS symptoms.

Once augmentation has resolved, patients can be prescribed a different drug (opioids or anticonvulsants) instead of a dopamine drug. Alternatively, they can take a different dopamine drug as a replacement. Developing augmentation with one drug does not always predict that it will occur with another. People often do not experience augmentation from the dopamine agonists after having this problem with a levodopa-containing drug. However, many experts have found that once augmentation has occurred with one dopamine agonist, it is more likely that people will suffer from this problem with another one. Therefore, physicians should proceed with caution when replacing one dopamine agonist with another after an episode of augmentation.

Unlike augmentation caused by drugs containing levodopa, which can cause severe problems, the augmentation from dopamine agonists is usually milder, and the drug may not need to be discontinued. RLS symptoms do not become as intense in augmentation from dopamine agonists, and symptom occurrence may shift to only a few hours earlier in the day. Treating these earlier symptoms may require people with RLS to take their medication earlier in the day or take an additional dose 1–2 hours before the symptoms occur. If people need increasingly higher doses to control symptoms, or if symptoms continue to shift to earlier in the day, people should replace the dopamine drug with another dopamine drug or with another class of drug.

The cause and mechanism of augmentation are not known. It is thought that the dopamine drugs may affect the dopamine receptors they act upon. The dopamine receptors may become downregulated (less responsive to the same amount of drug) and thus need more drug to produce the same effect. It is also possible that people produce less of their own dopamine in response to taking dopamine drugs. The decrease in their own naturally occurring dopamine may require replacement with higher doses of drugs. These explanations are similar to those thought to cause tolerance to a drug.

Short-acting dopamine agonists have a much higher risk of augmentation than do long-acting drugs. The reason for this phenomenon is also not understood, but one possibility is that the long-acting drugs cover up the worsening RLS symptoms better than the short-acting ones. So far, the long-acting drug cabergoline (half-life of over 65 hours) seems to have the lowest risk of augmentation; short-acting levodopa (half-life of 1.5–2 hours) has the highest risk. It is also puzzling why some people develop augmentation and others do not. This may be caused by biological differences. Studies have found that people without a family history of RLS may have a lower risk of developing augmentation.

> Dopamine drugs should be discontinued once severe augmentation has occurred and replaced with another type of medication, such as an opioid.

REBOUND

Rebound is often confused with augmentation. However, people with rebound develop early morning symptoms as opposed to augmentation, in which symptoms develop earlier in the evening or even in the afternoon. Rebound is considered an end-of-the dose effect. When the dose wears off, RLS symptoms start occurring at a time when they previously were not present. Therefore, this problem occurs only with short-acting drugs such as levodopa (half-life of 1.5–2 hours), which are effective for 3–4 hours, and rarely with the longer-acting drugs such as the dopamine agonists. However, dopamine drugs may cause rebound when people take their medication too early in the evening.

Studies with levodopa have found that rebound (20–24 percent) occurs less commonly than augmentation (up to 82 percent). Aside from being a morning problem, rebound is different from augmentation in several other ways. Rebound does not generally cause an increase in the intensity of RLS symptoms, which often occurs with augmentation, nor does it expand symptoms to other parts of the body.

Changing to a long-acting dopamine drug should reverse rebound. The longer-acting levodopa-containing drugs (Sinemet CR®, with a half-life of 4–6 hours) are less prone to cause rebound, and people taking dopamine agonists rarely complain of this problem. When rebound occurs as a result of taking a dopamine agonist too early in the evening, the dose can be increased or an additional dose can be taken right before going to bed. Some people prefer to take an extra dose of levodopa if symptoms bother them in the middle of the night. This may work well for those who experience rebound on an infrequent basis.

TOLERANCE

Tolerance is characterized by a decreased response to a drug over time, which then requires a higher dose to maintain the original effect. An increased need for a dopamine drug is often the result of tolerance; however, the natural progression of the RLS disorder itself must be ruled out as another possibility. It can be difficult to differentiate whether this increased need for medication is due to the development of tolerance or disease progression, because both processes tend to occur gradually over time. Generally, tolerance occurs at shorter time intervals and may require increasing the dose more frequently.

Tolerance is similar to augmentation in many ways, and some experts hypothesize that it may be a subtype of augmentation. Although the mechanisms for both these problems are not known, one theory is that they both may be due to downregulation of the dopamine receptors. Stopping a medication for a variable period of time will usually reestablish full effectiveness in both tolerance and augmentation.

In addition to being differentiated from the natural progression of RLS, tolerance must also be distinguished from augmentation, which can be difficult because tolerance actually meets two of the six features of augmentation (Table 8-1, Features 2 and 5). Tolerance can be distinguished from augmentation when the increase in RLS symptoms brought on by treatment exceeds the pretreatment level, because this only happens with augmentation. In addition, only augmentation has symptoms that occur earlier in the day or spread to other body parts.

Most physicians who treat RLS find tolerance to be a fairly common problem. Defining the exact frequency of tolerance is somewhat difficult, because there are not many long-term studies on RLS. Furthermore, tolerance may easily be confused with augmentation or with an increased need for drug from the natural progression of RLS. One study (Augmentation and Tolerance with Long-Term Pramipexole Treatment of RLS; 2004) found that tolerance developed in 46 percent of the people studied who were taking pramipexole.

Tolerance is usually not much of a problem compared to augmentation or rebound. Most physicians increase medication dosages when people complain that their medication is losing effectiveness. This usually solves the problem. Most people respond to modest increases in the dosage of a dopamine agonist. The study discussed above found that for those people with tolerance, the mean daily dose of pramipexole increased from 0.43 mg to 0.82 mg. If increasing the dose does not control symptoms, a change to another dopamine agonist may resolve the problem, because there is often no cross-tolerance from one dopamine agonist to another.

CHAPTER 9

Treating Secondary Restless Legs Syndrome and Patients with Additional Medical Problems

TREATMENT OF SECONDARY RLS

As DISCUSSED IN CHAPTER 3, secondary RLS occurs as the result of another medical condition. The three most common conditions that cause secondary RLS are pregnancy, end-stage renal disease (ESRD), and iron deficiency. When the conditions associated with secondary RLS are resolved, so generally are the RLS symptoms. Thus, diagnosing any underlying condition is important. Physicians and patients can then treat it, which, in turn, may resolve the RLS. Pregnancy, of course, is a condition that is not "treated." After delivery, however, the symptoms of RLS usually disappear within a few weeks, unless the woman had RLS before she became pregnant.

Iron Deficiency

Secondary RLS can be caused by a decrease in iron levels, and iron-replacement therapy may be helpful. Iron deficiency may make it harder for medications to relieve RLS. The most common reason for low iron levels is the loss of iron through blood loss that is not replaced adequately by dietary intake of iron. The two most common sources of blood loss are gastrointestinal (stomach or bowel) bleeding and menstrual blood loss in women. When serum iron levels are decreased, levels of transferrin (the protein that transports iron in the blood) are increased, but the amount of iron (percent iron saturation) attached to the transferrin is decreased. Serum ferritin (iron transport and storage protein) levels also decrease with iron deficiency.

RLS patients should have their serum ferritin levels determined by a blood test. This is a sensitive, accurate test for low iron levels. This test can determine low iron levels even when the more commonly performed serum iron level and percentage iron saturation tests are normal. Most labs report serum ferritin levels as normal if they are greater than 10 or 17 mcg/l, but studies have found that levels less than 50 mcg/l are associated with increased severity of RLS. When the serum ferritin level is less than 50 mcg/l, treatment with supplemental iron may relieve the symptoms of RLS.

This recommendation to consider iron therapy in people with serum ferritin levels greater than the lab normal of 10 or 17 mcg/l (but less than 50 mcg/l) may confuse physicians, especially when the usual blood tests for iron deficiency, serum iron, percentage iron saturation, and hemoglobin levels are all normal. However, there is a greater chance of improving RLS with iron therapy when initial ferritin levels are lower (18–30 mcg/l or less).

> Ferritin blood levels are increased when a person is sick, such as with the common cold; testing should be done when the patient is in his or her usual state of health in order for the test to be accurate.

Over-the-counter iron pills should not be taken without the direct supervision of a physician, because taking too much iron can lead to other medical problems, such as acquired *hemochromatosis*. The physician should continue to monitor iron levels during iron therapy, and if the serum ferritin level exceeds 200 mcg/l and the percent serum iron saturation (of transferrin) exceeds 50%, therapy should be discontinued, because excessive iron can cause damage to the liver, pancreas, heart, skin, and joints.

Oral iron therapy is the most common treatment for iron deficiency. Iron tablets are available over the counter as ferrous sulfate 325 mg (alternately labeled as "65 mg of elemental iron"), ferrous fumarate 200 mg (66 mg of elemental iron), or ferrous gluconate 325 mg (sometimes better tolerated, but it has only 38 mg of elemental iron). The recommended dose of ferrous sulfate is 325 mg, taken three times a day about 1 hour before meals or 2 hours after meals. To improve the absorption of iron, 100–200 mg of vitamin C can be taken at the same time. Iron tablets often cause abdominal discomfort (nausea, bloating, or pain) or constipation. Taking iron with food instead of on an empty stomach may lessen abdominal discomfort, but this also decreases iron absorption quite significantly. Sustained-release products cause much less stomach discomfort, but are much less effective for supplying iron. They are also more expensive.

Iron therapy should be monitored by blood testing every 3–4 months and continued until the ferritin level is greater than 45–60 mcg/l, at which point it can be discontinued. Periodic monitoring of serum ferritin levels is still necessary to ensure that levels do not decrease, especially if RLS symptoms worsen.

There are alternative ways of administering iron if oral iron therapy is not tolerated or does not adequately raise serum ferritin levels. Iron can be given by intramuscular injection or intravenously. Both of these methods have an increased risk of side effects and should be considered only when the iron deficiency is severe enough to cause significant anemia. Several research papers have demonstrated that intravenous iron may be a potent treatment for RLS, even when the RLS is severe.

Many people do not benefit from oral iron therapy, even when serum ferritin levels are brought to therapeutic levels (over 45–60 mcg/l). This may result from the iron not entering into the brain from the blood. The higher levels of iron provided by intravenous iron therapy may account for the much higher success rate, but some people do not even respond to this more aggressive treatment.

End Stage Renal Disease

End stage renal disease (ESRD) occurs when damage to the kidneys results in loss of normal kidney function. When the kidneys fail, they can no longer clear toxins and unwanted waste products from the body. These patients usually go on *dialysis* (mechanical filtration of the blood). Studies have shown prevalence rates of RLS in people with ESRD to be 17–70%, indicating that RLS is a common problem with this disease.

Reversing the condition causing RLS will usually resolve symptoms. Studies have shown that kidney transplantation, which reverses ERSD, also relieves associated RLS symptoms. If available and appropriate, this is clearly the best and most effective therapy for both the ESRD and RLS. For people who cannot have kidney transplants and must continue on dialysis, therapy for their RLS symptoms is actually quite similar to people with normal kidneys, with some exceptions. One mode of therapy for RLS that is unique to ESRD is the use of epoetin alfa (Procrit® or Epogen®), a synthetic form of erythropoietin.

Erythropoietin is a protein that the kidneys normally produce. It stimulates the production of oxygen-carrying red blood cells in the bone marrow. The damaged kidneys of people with ERSD do not produce adequate amounts of erythropoietin. Therefore, they cannot stimulate the bone marrow to manufacture enough red blood cells, which is part of the reason why these patients are anemic. Studies have demonstrated that administering epoetin alfa intravenously or subcutaneously helps anemia and the associated RLS. Anemia in ESRD is often due to iron deficiency. There are studies showing that intravenous iron therapy can often dramatically improve RLS in people with ESRD who cannot take or benefit from oral iron.

Secondary RLS in people with ESRD can be treated with the same drugs used for people with normal kidneys as long as some adjustments are made in the dosage. The kidneys metabolize opioids and gabapentin, so people with kidney failure should take lower doses of these drugs. Studies have demonstrated that levodopa is effective for RLS in people with ESRD, but augmentation is a frequent problem, which limits the use of this medication. One study found gabapentin to be superior to levodopa for people on dialysis. Another study found that one low dose (200–300 mg) of gabapentin given after dialysis relieved RLS symptoms.

The dopamine agonists are effective for RLS in people with ESRD. One study showed that ropinirole was more effective than levodopa. Ropinirole is preferred over pramipexole because the liver metabolizes it, whereas the kidneys metabolize pramipexole. This makes it more difficult for physicians to determine the dosage of pramipexole for these patients.

Physicians frequently prescribe benzodiazepines and nonbenzodiazepine sleeping pills for people on dialysis who have trouble sleeping due to RLS symptoms, but this use of these drugs has not yet been formally studied with clinical trials. Usually these medications do not need a significant dose adjustment when used for people with ESRD, because the kidneys do not metabolize these drugs.

Almost all people with kidney failure should be able to get relief from their RLS symptoms with the proper use of the currently available medications. People with ESRD should not settle for less and suffer from RLS, because there are several treatment options available. It is important to work closely with the nephrologist (kidney specialist) who is managing the patient's kidney failure. The nephrologist will know how to adjust the dosage of the RLS medications that the kidneys can no longer metabolize.

TREATMENT OF RLS IN PEOPLE WITH PSYCHIATRIC CONDITIONS

Although the treatment options for RLS are similar for everyone, some groups of people require special considerations. Physicians should treat every RLS patient as an individual and devise a unique plan based on their needs and other health issues. Treating people with RLS who have psychiatric disorders can present significant challenges. The primary concern is that most of the psychiatric medications tend to worsen RLS. People with psychiatric diseases generally tolerate RLS medications well. Therefore, physicians can prescribe them according to the RLS treatment algorithms discussed in Chapters 5, 6, and 7.

Depression and Anxiety

Studies have found that depression and anxiety are much more common in people with RLS than in the general population. Untreated RLS symptoms can easily provoke or worsen these problems. Furthermore, many of the drugs used to treat these disorders exacerbate RLS symptoms. Physicians must recognize these common problems in people with RLS and treat them carefully.

Depression and anxiety can occur separately, but they most often occur together. In addition, many of the medications that help depression also improve problems with anxiety. Physicians treat people who only have anxiety with the same antidepressant medications as those with depression. However, anxious people also benefit from many of the benzodiazepine sedatives listed in Table 5-1. These sedatives help people with RLS get to sleep.

One of the first concerns when assessing treatment needs is to establish whether the depression or anxiety is actually a separate problem, or whether it is caused by years of untreated significant RLS symptoms. People with moderate to severe RLS who have been undiagnosed for many years can develop anxiety and depression. Their "anxious legs or arms" can easily spread to a generalized feeling of anxiety. Many people complain about increasing anxiety when they anticipate another night of walking instead of sleeping. The lack of sleep results in disruption of their daily life, producing depression. For these people, simply treating their RLS symptoms satisfactorily may resolve their anxiety or depression problems.

> In the past, I was diagnosed with everything from schizophrenia to depression to anxiety disorders; you name it. But a few months ago, after having an accident where I fell down some steps, a friend of mine gave me a dose of hydrocodone. I never experienced anything more amazing in my life. The restlessness in the legs disappeared, and with it also went the anxiety, depression, and irritability—all the general misery I've experienced all my life.
>
> The conclusion now is very, very clear: there is one problem, and one only, from which the rest of my problems derive. When the RLS is eliminated, the level of my efficiency, the height of my mood, the strength of my concentration, my natural gregariousness all come out; ME, in other words!
>
> DAN HOBBS

Before attributing anxiety or depression to RLS, it must be ascertained that these problems occurred after the RLS symptoms disrupted a person's life. As RLS progresses over many years or decades, it may be difficult to sort out when the depression and anxiety started in relation to the onset of disruptive RLS symptoms. Physicians who have patients with untreated anxiety or depression—who have also not had their RLS treated yet—should first treat the RLS and then see if the depression or anxiety resolves. Once they alleviate the RLS symptoms, it should be clear whether the patient still has depression or anxiety that needs treatment.

Physicians often prescribe antidepressants for people with untreated RLS and must decide whether to continue the medication after they have treated the RLS symptoms successfully. This can be a difficult decision. Once the RLS has been resolved, it may be reasonable to taper the depression or anxiety medications slowly. If this process precipitates worsening depression or anxiety, the medications can be started again.

People with RLS who clearly have a separate psychiatric disorder and are benefiting from psychiatric drugs should remain on those medications. Physicians may have a difficult decision to make if they suspect the psychiatric medication is worsening the RLS. In this case, it may be reasonable to substitute a medication that does not produce side effects.

Most of the drugs that treat depression and anxiety worsen RLS; however, some antidepressant drugs do not (see Table 4-9). Bupropion and trazodone are probably the best choices among the RLS-friendly antidepressants, followed by the secondary amine tricyclics (desipramine). These drugs are not always effective for every patient with depression and anxiety, so physicians often need to use the less RLS-friendly drugs. People may experience fewer problems with the RLS-unfriendly antidepressants if they take them at lower doses or in combination with the RLS-friendly drugs.

Not all of the drugs listed in Tables 4-7, 4-8, and 4-9 cause worsening of RLS in every patient. Many people notice no change in their symptoms with these medications, or they may even experience improvement. The reason for the variability of this response is not well understood. Anxiety can worsen RLS symptoms, so perhaps by lessening anxiety, these medications may indirectly relieve RLS.

It can be difficult to change a psychiatric medication that is controlling significant anxiety or depression. However, changing medication may result in better control of RLS symptoms or a decrease in the dosage of the RLS medications. This benefit must be weighed against the possibility that significant depression or anxiety may return and cause distress. In addition, it usually takes a few weeks for a new medication to be effective in alleviating depression or anxiety. Therefore, before embarking upon the search for a more RLS-friendly drug, the patient should consider all the pros and cons and discuss the situation with their psychiatric and RLS physicians.

Schizophrenia and Bipolar Disorder (Manic Depression)

The neuroleptic medications used to treat schizophrenia and bipolar disorder usually block dopamine receptors, which typically worsens RLS (see Table 4-10). However, changing or stopping these medications can result in major relapses in otherwise stable people. Schizophrenia and bipolar disorder are serious illnesses, and treatment should continue even when the medications are clearly worsening RLS symptoms.

At the time of this writing, there is only one neuroleptic medication that is RLS friendly: aripiprazole (Abilify®). This drug has dopamine agonist properties, which may account for its positive effect on RLS. Despite the lack of any scientific studies on the use of this drug in RLS, many people have reported that aripiprazole has relieved their RLS symptoms. Aripiprazole may be a good choice when physicians need to start or add a neuroleptic drug.

Pregnancy and Breastfeeding with RLS

Pregnancy

As discussed in Chapter 3, RLS during pregnancy is common. Women with a family history of RLS often have their first experience with this disorder during pregnancy. Symptoms may start or worsen early in the pregnancy, but the third trimester is usually the worst time for most pregnant women with RLS. Although symptoms may be mild, many pregnant women suffer from intense, bothersome symptoms. This is especially true for women with preexisting RLS.

As soon as I became pregnant, I started to get a severe case of RLS where it lasts all night and is very painful. I have to keep moving, which is exhausting when you're pregnant. I went to my local doctor in tears, as I would fall asleep at around 5 a.m. and then get up to go to work at 7 A.M.

My doctor said there was nothing I could do about it during pregnancy, so I tried to cope with the pain and lack of sleep. I eventually broke down and ended up in the hospital due to exhaustion, major sleep deprivation, depression, hallucinations, and dangerous driving. I even had to quit work.

TINA HARRISON, Australia

Nondrug therapy may suffice for pregnant women who develop mild RLS symptoms. Avoiding medications is always one of the main goals. However, when symptoms are not controlled, or are severe or disruptive, pregnant women should consider treatment with medication. Iron, folate, and magnesium are safe and may be helpful for pregnant women with RLS; however, no benefit has yet been proven. Studies show that low iron levels increase a pregnant woman's risk of having RLS, but they have not yet demonstrated that taking iron relieves RLS. Furthermore, if low iron levels are causing the RLS symptoms, why do these symptoms resolve within a few weeks of delivery, which is too short a time to increase iron levels, especially considering the increased blood loss during delivery?

There have been a few studies indicating that low levels of folate or magnesium may be associated with RLS in pregnancy. However, the evidence so far does not show any benefit from treating pregnant women with RLS with these supplements. Nevertheless, if ferritin or folate levels are low in pregnant women with RLS, supplementation is a safe and reasonable course of action, whether or not it results in improvement of RLS symptoms.

Physicians must choose medications for pregnant women carefully in order to minimize the risk of fetal abnormalities. There is little research and few guidelines on the treatment of RLS in pregnancy. Therefore, most RLS specialists prescribe only those drugs that are both safe for pregnant women and effective for RLS. They may also use these drugs in a more limited fashion.

Table 9-1 FDA Risk Categories of RLS Drugs for Use in Pregnant Women

Pregnancy risk category	Drug name
A	None
B	Cabergoline, pergolide (but limited data), zolpidem, methadone (low dose), oxycodone (short-term use)
C	Pramipexole, ropinirole, levodopa, clonidine, zaleplon, eszopiclone, carbamazepine, gabapentin, propoxyphene, codeine, hydrocodone, all for short-term use, fentanyl, hydromorphone, morphine, Demerol®, levorphanol, tramadol
D	Alprazolam, clonazepam, and most benzodiazepine sedatives, propoxyphene, codeine, hydrocodone, oxycodone, all for long-term use, methadone (higher doses)
X	Temazepam

Table 9-1 lists the commonly used RLS medications and their safety for pregnancy. Category A drugs are considered completely safe during pregnancy; Category X drugs have the highest risk of damaging the developing fetus. Physicians prescribe Category B drugs commonly during pregnancy, but with caution. Category C drugs are considerably more risky during pregnancy, and physicians should only prescribe them under extreme circumstances and after serious consideration of their risks and benefits. Category D drugs are rarely used, and pregnant women should avoid Category X drugs entirely. Note that iron and folate are in Category A, and magnesium is in Category B

There are no Category A drugs for RLS, and cabergoline (Dostinex®) and pergolide (Permax®) are the only Category B dopamine agonists. There are limited data available on pergolide because few studies have been done on this drug for use in pregnancy. There is more extensive evidence to show that cabergoline is reasonably safe during pregnancy; however, it is usually prohibitively expensive.

Narcotics are a common choice for treating pregnant women with severe RLS. Methadone in low doses or oxycodone for short-term treatment can be effective. There are considerable data on the use of methadone during pregnancy. Narcotics must be stopped late in the pregnancy because they have been associated with neonatal withdrawal syndrome and respiratory depression. When RLS causes severe insomnia in pregnant women, zolpidem (Ambien®) is a reasonable choice because it is a Category B drug.

> The Category B drugs, including methadone, oxycodone, cabergoline, and zolpidem, are the safest drugs to treat RLS in pregnant women.

To keep the risk of developing fetal abnormalities as low as possible, pregnant women with RLS should take narcotics at the lowest effective dose and for the shortest possible time, although this may result in less-than-optimum treatment. The information on the use of drugs in pregnancy is always changing. Pregnant women should check with their personal obstetrician before taking any medication. In addition, the following Web sites can be searched for the most current information on medicines that are safe for use during pregnancy: www.motherisk.org; www.perinatology.com; and http://orpheus.ucsd.edu/ctis/.

Breastfeeding

The concerns about drugs taken by breastfeeding women include (1) the affect on the mother's ability to nurse and (2) the effect on the child receiving the breast milk. Before taking any medication, a nursing mother should always check with her pediatrician to be certain that the drug will not harm her child.

The dopamine agonists (see Table 5-4) are all unsuitable for nursing mothers. They inhibit the secretion of prolactin, which, in turn, decreases the production of breast milk. Most narcotics (see Table 5-3) and tramadol either enter into the breast milk in significant amounts or have not been studied well enough in nursing mothers to be considered safe. However, methadone has been evaluated adequately in pregnancy and is considered safe for use by nursing mothers because it passes only minimally into breast milk.

> Methadone is the safest drug to treat RLS in nursing mothers.

Gabapentine passes into breast milk, but its effect on nursing infants is unknown, and its use by nursing women is not recommended. The other anticonvulsant drugs listed in Table 6-1 are also not recommended for use by nursing mothers.

The benzodiazepines (see Table 5-1) are all excreted in breast milk and can cause infants to become lethargic and lose weight. They are clearly not recommended for use in nursing mothers. Similarly, the non-benzodiazepine sleeping pills (see Table 5-2) also transfer into breast milk and are not recommended for mothers who breastfeed their infants.

RLS AND SURGICAL PATIENTS

Surgery is especially frightening for people with RLS. Not only do they have to face the usual concerns of the risks of surgery and postoperative pain, they also have worry about whether their RLS symptoms will be adequately controlled. Different problems arise depending on whether patients have their surgery performed under local or general anesthesia.

Patients are usually awake, or somewhat drowsy but not asleep, when local anesthesia is used. Oral intake of medications is usually stopped the night before surgery, including those for RLS. Therefore, people undergoing surgery with local anesthesia are likely to develop RLS symptoms during surgery. They may not be able to remain immobile, which may interfere with the procedure. This possibility should be discussed with the physician prior to surgery so a plan can be developed to prevent RLS symptoms during surgery.

Some physicians allow surgical patients to take their RLS medications a few hours before surgery with just a sip of water. If this is not appropriate, the physician can give the patient an injection of a narcotic before surgery. This can be repeated during or after surgery if the RLS symptoms become active again. Patients who must remain confined to a hospital bed for prolonged periods postoperatively can also experience the symptoms of RLS. PLM that occurs during local anesthesia can be disruptive to surgery, but can be resolved with a narcotic injection. PLM may also occur in patients receiving epidural or spinal anesthesia, which can also require an injection of a narcotic.

Narcotic injections are often part of the preoperative medications given to patients receiving local anesthesia. These injections should prevent RLS symptoms from occurring during the procedure. Unfortunately, physicians often give antiemetic/nausea drugs (see Table 4-5) before surgery, which tend to worsen RLS. Most surgeons and anesthesiologists are not aware of RLS and the drugs that worsen it, and patients should give their physicians a list of these possibly problematic drugs and the alternatives well in advance of any surgery.

RLS is not a problem during general anesthesia because the patient is asleep and unconscious, and a person must be awake to perceive abnormal sensations and the urge to move. PLMS should not be a problem because most often the patient is paralyzed by the anesthesia, which prevents leg jerks. Once the surgery is completed and general anesthesia is ended, RLS symptoms may become active again. Most surgical procedures result in significant postoperative pain, and high-potency narcotic injections are commonly given to control it. These narcotic injections should also control any RLS symptoms that occur during the immediate postoperative period. An alternative to narcotic injections postoperative for those who cannot take oral medications is the Parkinson's disease injectable drug apomorphine (Apokyn®). This drug is a D1, D2 receptor agonist, meaning it acts on the dopamine type 1 and 2 receptors. It does not contain morphine and is not a narcotic.

Usually within 1–3 days following surgery, physicians will attempt to discontinue narcotic medication, although this might take much longer with surgeries causing significant postoperative pain. As soon as the physician allows oral intake (usually within a day or so), RLS medications can be resumed, although this can be delayed after abdominal surgery. People who are sedentary after surgery (such as after orthopedic procedures) may need to increase the dosage of their RLS medications. In addition, surgery or any other trauma to the body can worsen RLS and may require an increased level of RLS medication. Narcotics, given as needed, may be a reasonable choice until the person with RLS can ambulate and symptoms decrease.

Postoperative nausea, which is quite common, can be problematic because almost all the medications used to treat it tend to worsen RLS (see Table 4-4). Alternatives include the antinausea medications listed in Table 4-5. Patients should make their surgeons and other treating physicians aware of these drugs well in advance of any surgery and review the entire list of medications that worsen RLS, which should prevent inadvertent use that can exacerbate RLS symptoms during or after surgery.

Patients who are on opioids should also avoid opioid antagonists such as naloxone, naltrexone, and Talwin NX®. With proper planning and care, people with RLS should not fear surgery for its potential to worsen their symptoms. Physicians should be able to prevent or control RLS symptoms during and after surgery if they are made aware of the possible difficulties.

CHAPTER 10

What About Treating Periodic Limb Movement Disorder?

People with PLMD often feel that their problem does not get much attention. Even in this book, discussion about RLS far exceeds that of PLMD. The reason for this discrepancy is that a controversy exists about whether or not PLMD is a real disorder. Sleep specialists are divided as to what constitutes PLMD and when, or if, it should be treated. Before physicians treat a medical condition they must be certain that the disorder is causing a significant medical problem and that treating it will resolve the problem. Many of the people who go to their doctor complaining of PLMD also have RLS. In this case the choice to treat PLMD is easy, because the drugs used for RLS also help PLMD. However, many physicians have difficulty deciding how or whether to treat people with PLMD who do not have RLS.

For the purposes of treatment, PLM can be divided into two groups: PLM that disturb the bed partner but not the patient, and PLM that disturb the patient.

PLM That Disturbs the Bed Partner but Not the Patient

A person may have hundreds of PLM throughout the night; however, if these leg kicks do not cause sleep arousals (changes from deeper sleep to lighter sleep) or awakenings, they usually have no impact on the person's health. If the person has no complaints of daytime fatigue or sleepiness, the leg jerks are merely a curiosity or, at worst, bothersome to the bed partner. This type of person does not have PLMD and may not need drug treatment.

Bed partners of these nighttime kickers may complain bitterly about their sleep being disturbed by numerous and occasionally vigorous leg jerks. This can cause considerable disharmony and conflict in a relationship. The sleep-deprived bed partner may demand that the PLM patient leave the bed. Sleeping in separate rooms will solve this problem, but this is often an unacceptable solution for couples who value sleeping together.

There is a somewhat better solution, which is to change to twin beds. The twin beds can even be made up with one bed sheet. If the leg kicks are so vigorous that they still disturb the bed partner, separating the beds by about one inch should resolve this problem. A king-sized bed with a memory foam mattress is another useful alternative that allows the couple to sleep as far apart as possible. Tempur-Pedic® is one of the more popular brands of memory foam mattresses, but there are several others. Some of these contain foam that is less dense, which does not absorb movement vibrations as well. These mattresses are usually cheaper and not as firm. Although this is a second choice to twin beds, memory foam is effective at dampening vibrations caused by leg kicks. People and their bed partners should try these beds before buying one to assess the bed's comfort and ability to diminish the vibrations from leg kicks. Although many people find memory foam mattresses comfortable, others may find that they do not sleep well on them and that they are too warm. Another concern is that some people may be very allergic to the memory foam. It is advisable to buy a bed that provides a home trial period with a moneyback guarantee.

These bed solutions may solve the problem for many couples; however, they may not work for couples who find it unacceptable to sleep without snuggling close together. This can be difficult. Taking medication is the only certain solution to preventing people with PLMS from kicking their bed partners. Most physicians feel uncomfortable prescribing medications for symptoms that do not directly affect the patient. Some people with PLMS may warrant treatment if they experience enough emotional difficulty because they cannot sleep cuddled up to their bed partner. These cases should be decided on an individual basis, with drugs chosen from the options discussed below.

PLM That Disturb the Patient

It has been difficult to prove that the sleep arousals from PLMS result in daytime fatigue or sleepiness. People with PLMS often have other diseases that can cause daytime fatigue or sleepiness, such as RLS or sleep apnea. The studies done so far have not definitively proven that frequent PLM arousals cause daytime problems and that treating the PLMS improves these problems. In fact, one study found that there was no relationship between the PLM arousal index and subjective complaints of disturbed sleep, an objective measure of daytime sleepiness, or a sense of awakening refreshed in the morning.

Most physicians will consider treating people who have documented PLM that prevent them from falling asleep or wake them up frequently enough to cause significant insomnia. This certainly would qualify as a true disorder and warrant a diagnosis of PLMD. Many physicians will also treat people with frequent PLM arousals (usually more than 25 per hour documented by a sleep study) and significant daytime fatigue or sleepiness that is not a result of any other apparent cause.

Drugs Used to Treat PLMD

Most of the drugs used to treat RLS also can be used totreat PLMD. Some of these drugs decrease the number of leg kicks; others just decrease the number of arousals from the leg kicks.

Dopamine Drugs

The dopamine agonists (see Table 5-4) are the best studied drugs for PLMS. Studies have shown that many of these drugs decrease PLMS; most of them also decrease PLM-associated arousals and awakenings. They are usually the first choice of therapy for both daily RLS and PLMD. Medications containing levodopa also help PLMS. They can be taken at lower doses than those used to treat RLS, and thus have less of a tendency to cause augmentation. However, some people with PLMD who are treated with dopamine drugs may develop waking symptoms of RLS.

Benzodiazepine Sedative/Hypnotic Drugs

Benzodiazepine (see Table 5-1) sedatives and hypnotics may reduce the amount of PLM somewhat, but they are better at reducing the arousals and awakenings that occur from leg kicks. Most studies have been done on clonazepam, which is a long-acting drug. Care should be taken with the longer-acting benzodiazepines, because although they reduce the disruption of sleep by PLM, they may cause daytime fatigue or sleepiness.

Opioids (Narcotics)

There are only a few studies showing the effect of opioids (see Table 5-3) on PLMS. Some studies, mostly using propoxyphene and oxycodone, show that the number of PLM are reduced; others show that just the arousals from the PLM are decreased.

Anticonvulsants

Few studies have been done examining the effect of anticonvulsants other than gabapentin (see Table 6-1) on PLMS. Most of the studies with these drugs have been of RLS symptoms and have not included sleep studies, which are necessary to analyze the effects on PLMS. One study found that carbamazepine did not improve PLMS. Several studies have found that gabapentin reduces PLMS, and many people have reported positive results with this drug. All of the other anticonvulsants may be useful for PLMS, but so far evidence exists only for lamotrigine, valproate, and probably levetiracetam.

Melatonin

One study of people with PLMD who did not have RLS found that melatonin at 3 mg decreased PLM and PLM arousals. There is little other experience with this drug for treating PLMD. In addition, the long-term effects of using melatonin are not known.

Treating PLMD with Medication

Treating people who have both RLS and PLMD is relatively easy because the treatment for RLS will usually resolve PLMD. However, people with isolated PLMD may be more problematic to treat. When treating PLMD, it is necessary to monitor the effect of the therapy. People with PLMD can be divided into two groups based on the methods necessary to check the effectiveness of treatment.

The first group consists of those people who are aware of their PLM and can report to their physician when the treatment has been successful. These people have PLM that prevent them from falling asleep or wake them up in the middle of the night. This also applies to people who do not have PLMD, but who are being treated to prevent their legs kicks from bothering their bed partners. In this case, the bed partners can easily report when therapy is successful.

The second group consists of people who are unaware of their PLM and cannot directly report on the results of therapy. Most people are unaware of their PLM because the PLM do not wake them up, but rather cause sleep arousals that they cannot perceive. Frequent PLM-associated sleep arousals may result in daytime sleepiness or fatigue. Although the effectiveness of treatment can be assessed by its effect on the daytime complaints, there may not always be a direct correlation between these two concerns.

Ideally, a repeat sleep study would be helpful to monitor the effect on sleep after each dosage change of the drug being used to treat PLM. Physicians could then determine whether the drug has decreased PLMS and sleep arousals from leg kicks. This, of course, is impractical, because sleep studies are expensive and time-consuming. *Actigraphy* is an alternative to monitoring PLM with an overnight sleep study. It can be done at home, with the patient wearing an actigraph on each ankle—this is a device that looks much like a wrist watch and contains a motion sensor. The actigraph detects leg movements and is as accurate as a sleep study in determining the number of PLMS. The data can be downloaded into a computer and analyzed. This may be a reasonable way to monitor therapy, in addition to the patient's subjective improvement of daytime complaints, to see if the medication is improving the PLMS. However, actigraphy only gives information about changes in the number of PLMS, not the sleep arousals caused by them.

Dopamine agonists, benzodiazepines, and gabapentin improve PLMD.

Dopamine drugs are usually the first choice for treating PLMD. These drugs should be started at the lowest dose, taken about 1–2 hours before bedtime. The dose can be increased slowly until treatment goals have been met. If dopamine drugs are not tolerated or are not fully effective, benzodiazepines can be substituted or added. Even if the benzodiazepines do not decrease the number of leg movements, they will decrease arousals and usually result in increased sleep time. This may be the reason that these patients feel better during the daytime. Studies have shown gabapentin to be effective, so it is also a reasonable choice. There is not much evidence demonstrating the effectiveness of opioids for PLMS, and they are generally not used for this problem.

CHAPTER 11

Restless Legs Syndrome in Children

CLINICAL MANIFESTATIONS

Sam G. is an 8-year-old boy who was reported by his teachers in school to be fidgety, restless, irritable, moody, and easily distractible in class. One of his teachers has repeatedly sent him to the school principal's office for discipline due to his nonattention and angry disposition. Sam's concerned parents noticed that he was not sleeping well and his bad behavior at school was even worse at home, where he frequently had tantrums. His parents considered taking Sam to see a child psychiatrist, but the school nurse suggested they first make an appointment with Sam's pediatrician. He was diagnosed with attention deficit–hyperactivity disorder (ADHD) and prescribed Ritalin®. Sam's parents and teachers noticed no change in his behavior after one month on Ritalin®, and he was referred to a pediatric neurologist who diagnosed RLS and started him on a low dose of ropinirole. Sam's condition improved within 2 weeks to the point that he was attentive and pleasant during class and his disruptive behavior and grades markedly improved.

Sam's case is a fairly typical manifestation of RLS in children, and any child with similar symptoms should be evaluated for RLS. The challenge in diagnosing children with RLS is that they are often inaccurate or poor historians. They sometimes minimize their symptoms to avoid visiting the physician. Nevertheless, the history remains the most important element in making a diagnosis in a child suspected of having RLS or PLMD. Many children who suffer from these conditions are low in iron and, as with adults, measurement of serum ferritin is important.

> The challenge in diagnosing children with RLS is that they are often inaccurate or poor historians.

The American Academy of Sleep Medicine criteria for the diagnosis of RLS in children (age 2–12 years) are listed in Table 11-1. The criteria for the diagnosis of probable and possible RLS in children—as developed by the participants in the Restless Legs Syndrome Diagnosis and Epidemiology Workshop at the National Institutes of Health on May 1–3, 2002, in collaboration with members of the International Restless Legs Syndrome Study Group—are listed in Tables 11-2 and 11-3, respectively. If the child is suspected of having PLMD, the criteria listed in Table 11-4 can be used to diagnose PLMD.

Table 11-1   Criteria for the Diagnosis of RLS in Children (2–12 Years)

(A alone, or B and C satisfy the criteria.)

A. The child meets all four essential adult criteria for RLS (see Table 2-1 on page 21) and relates a description in his or her own words that is consistent with leg discomfort. The child may use terms such as *oowies, tickle, spiders, boo-boos, want to run,* and *a lot of energy in my legs* to describe symptoms. Age-appropriate descriptors are encouraged.

OR

B. The child meets all four essential adult criteria for RLS (see Table 2-1 on page 21) but does not relate a description in his or her own words that is consistent with leg discomfort.

AND

C. The child has at least two of the following three findings:
   a. Sleep disturbance for age.
   b. A biological parent or sibling with definite RLS.
   c. A documented (by polysomnogram or sleep study) periodic limb movement index of five or more movements per hour of sleep.

Table 11-2 Criteria for the Diagnosis of *Probable* RLS in Children

1. The child meets all essential adult criteria for RLS, except criterion number 4 (the urge to move or sensations are worse in the evening or at night than during the day).

AND

2. The child has a biologic parent or sibling with definite RLS.

OR*

1. The child is observed to have behavior manifestations of lower-extremity discomfort when sitting or lying accompanied by motor movement of the affected limbs, the discomfort has characteristics of adult criteria 2, 3, and 4 (worse during rest and inactivity, relieved by movement, and worse during the evening and at night).

AND

2. The child has a biologic parent or sibling with definite RLS.

---

* This last probable category is intended for young children or cognitively impaired children who do not have sufficient language to describe the sensory component of RLS.

Table 11-3 Criteria for the Diagnosis of *Possible* RLS in Children

1. The child has periodic limb movement disorder.

AND

2. The child has a biologic parent or sibling with definite RLS, but the child does not meet definite or probable childhood RLS definitions.

Table 11-4 Criteria for the Diagnosis of PLMD in Children

A. Polysomnography demonstrates repetitive, highly stereotyped limb movements that are:

   a. 0.5–5 seconds in duration.

   b. Of amplitude greater than or equal to 25 percent of toe dorsiflexion during calibration.

   c. In a sequence of four or more movements.

   d. Separated by an interval of more than 5 seconds (from limb-movement onset to limb-movement onset) and less than 90 seconds (typically there is an interval of 20–40 seconds).

B. The PLMS Index exceeds five per hour in children.

C. There is clinical sleep disturbance or a complaint of daytime fatigue.

D. The PLM are not better explained by another current sleep disorder, medical or neurological disorder, mental disorder, medication use, or substance use disorder; for example, the PLM at the termination of cyclically occurring apneas should not be counted as true PLMS or PLMD.

When children with symptoms of RLS or PLMD are evaluated by a clinician, they may be diagnosed with "growing pains" or ADHD, as in Sam's case. These conditions, as well as others, may be differentiated from RLS or PLMD by a number of symptoms.

Growing Pains

This condition may be difficult to differentiate from RLS because of the overlap of symptoms and because RLS may be an aspect of growing pains. Typical symptoms include throbbing or painful legs before falling asleep or while awaking from sleep. Growing pains generally occur in early-to-late childhood, with symptoms that are most prominent in the muscles, often in the front of the thighs, calves, or behind the knees. Similar to RLS, there does appear to be a circadian variation to the symptoms, with appearance of the symptoms typically in the late afternoon to bedtime. Unlike RLS, the urge to move or unpleasant sensations are generally not partially or totally relieved by movement. However, the condition does tend to respond to massage, ice packs and warm compresses, and acetaminophen or ibuprofen.

ADHD

The exact relationship between RLS, PLMD, and ADHD is unknown. However, there does appear to be a relationship among these disorders because of the fact that RLS and PLMD are common in children with ADHD; ADHD is common in children with RLS and PLMD; both RLS and ADHD are characterized by motor restlessness; both RLS and ADHD demonstrate dopaminergic deficits on brain-imaging studies; and RLS, PLMD, and ADHD respond to dopaminergic agents. Complicating the relationships among these disorders is the fact that RLS is frequently mistaken for ADHD, as in the case of Sam G. Given this overlap of ADHD with RLS and PLMD, a child suspected of having symptoms of one or more of these disorders needs to be carefully evaluated by a pediatric neurologist or sleep specialist.

How best to treat children with ADHD and either RLS or PLMD remains an open question. Stimulants such as modafinil or methylphenidate may improve daytime symptoms, and typical treatments for RLS may ease sleep complaints. Improving sleep can, in turn, reduce the problems of ADHD. The course of treatment can be decided by a specialist, with the best results being obtained through trial and error.

Muscle Pains

This condition is typically related to overuse or exertion and may be differentiated from RLS in that the former condition is more cramp-like or painful in quality, temporally related to strenuous activity, and not easily relieved by movement of the affected leg(s). Rest and alternation of ice packs and warm compresses typically help relieve the condition.

Leg Cramps

This condition is difficult to distinguish from RLS, even in adults. However, the main distinguishing features are that leg cramps typically affect one leg, are restricted to a specific muscle group or groups, are more painful, and are not easily relieved by movement of the affected leg. Checking the electrolytes in the blood for an ionic imbalance (electrolytes include sodium, calcium, and potassium) may be prudent in severe cases, but most cramps respond to rest and alternating of ice packs and warm compresses.

Osgood-Schlatter's Disease

This condition represents a common cause of knee pain in a growing child, typically between the ages of 10 and 14 years. Osgood-Schlatter's disease is caused by injury to a growth plate in the front of the knee. This condition can be distinguished from RLS because, in addition to pain, tenderness, and swelling, it is frequently associated with strenuous activity, such as sports and bicycling. The suspected etiology for Osgood-Schlatter's is an abnormal strain of the patellar tendon, which results in pain at the site of attachment at the kneecap. Treatment consists of the avoidance of activities that require excessive kneeling or movement of the knee, which can aggravate the condition. Alternating ice packs with warm compresses and acetaminophen or ibuprofen may provide temporary relief. If the condition persists, an orthopedist may prescribe a custom-fitted shoe insert (an orthotic) that can correct any problem in foot position, which, in turn, may result in the abnormal knee function seen in Osgood-Schlatter's disease.

Chondromalacia Patella

This condition is a frequently the result of poor movement of the patella (kneecap) femoral joint, which causes damage to the underside of the patella. Chrondomalacia patella is distinguishable from RLS in that (1) it is frequently characterized by pain at the knee joint, (2) movement of the leg exacerbates rather than relieves the pain, and (3) it is typically related to overuse or strain of the joint caused by exercise or sports. It can be treated by rest, anti-inflammatory drugs, and orthopedist-prescribed muscle-strengthening exercises and orthotics.

Arthralgias (Joint Aches)

This group of conditions can be symptomatic of any number of various disorders that may result in joint pain, ranging from Lyme disease to juvenile rheumatoid arthritis. Arthralgias can be differentiated from RLS in that they are characterized by pain and restricted to a specific joint or joints. Unlike RLS, swelling and tenderness may also be present at the affected joint(s) and the discomfort is made worse by activity rather than better. Joint pain not related to sports or exercise should be evaluated by a pediatrician, particularly if the pain is persistent.

Obstructive Sleep Apnea and PLMD

A sleep-related breathing disorder, such as obstructive sleep apnea, can produce daytime symptoms, including lack of concentration, irritability, mood changes, and restlessness, which are identical to those of RLS. In obstructive sleep apnea, the upper airway collapses repetitively during sleep, resulting in breathing pauses. These pauses eventually cause brief awakenings that allow the normal breathing pattern to resume. The awakenings result in disturbed, fragmented sleep, which, in turn, causes daytime symptoms. Obstructive sleep apnea can be differentiated from RLS by the symptoms of snoring, noisy breathing, or witnessed breathing pauses during sleep and, most importantly, by an overnight sleep study.

The child may also have limb movements that occur at the end of an apnea or breathing pause; these should not be interpreted as PLM because they may represent a response to the abnormal breathing event. In addition, if the child is suspected of having PLMD, the sleep study criteria in Table 11-4 can be used to diagnose PLMD. Data obtained from a sleep study will enable the clinician to diagnose obstructive sleep apnea. A tonsillectomy and adenoidectomy can result in a cure in more than 90 percent of the cases. Continuous positive airway pressure (CPAP) is another treatment choice.

TREATMENT

There have been no randomized placebo-controlled trials for the treatment of RLS or PLMD in children. In fact, the *Practice Parameters for the Treatment of Restless Legs Syndrome and Periodic Limb Movement Disorder*, published in 1999 by the Standards of Practice Committee of the American Academy of Sleep Medicine, states: "No specific recommendations can be made regarding treatment of children with RLS and PLMD." Further, it states, "The benzodiazepines, anticonvulsants, alpha-adrenergic, and opioid classes of medication have been used widely in children for treatment of other medical disorders, but no acceptable trials have been performed in children with RLS or PLMD." Since there are no FDA-approved medications for the treatment of RLS or PLMD in children, the risks of treating children for these conditions with the existing medications are unknown.

The ultimate goal of any treatment for RLS and PLMD in children is to improve daytime function by improving the quality and quantity of sleep. This entails improving the sleepiness, hyperactivity, mood, restlessness, and distractibility that are symptomatic of RLS or PLMD in children. Controlling the leg discomfort of RLS is important, particularly if it is severe and directly results in the impairment of daytime function. Referral to a pediatric neurologist or sleep specialist is recommended for the management of childhood RLS or PLMD.

> The first step in the treatment of RLS in children is the maintenance of good sleep habits.

The first step in the treatment of RLS in children is the maintenance of good sleep habits. The child often experiences delays in going to sleep and morning awakenings, which are worsened by the leg discomfort of RLS. A strict bedtime and morning rise time schedule should be followed. The child should be exposed to bright light—in the form of morning sunlight or from a light box—beginning within a few minutes of awakening and lasting for at least half an hour. Bright light within a few hours of bedtime should be avoided because it can delay the onset of sleep. Bedtime rituals, such as reading a bedtime story to the child and having a glass of warm milk, should be consistently followed on a nightly basis. The child should not watch television or play computer games within 1–2 hours of bedtime. Caffeinated soft drinks should be avoided from the afternoon up to bedtime, and any exercise or heavy snacks should be avoided near bedtime. SSRIs can cause RLS or PLMD in children, and changing to another class of antidepressants, such as bupropion, is recommended in these cases.

The long-term use of medications for the treatment of RLS or PLMD in children has not been studied, and the effects of RLS medications over time are unknown; thus, caution should be exercised. Clonazepam and clonidine have been studied in children with RLS, and both are fairly well tolerated, although it is prudent to have the child first be seen by a sleep specialist if the child has symptoms of obstructive sleep apnea, including snoring, breathing pauses, daytime sleepiness, or hyperactivity. Clonazepam can worsen sleep apnea by relaxing the upper airway muscles, which increases the frequency and severity of apnea episodes during the night. Clonidine can induce nightmares in some children. Dopaminergic medications are well tolerated, but up to 20 percent of children taking levodopa/carbidopa may develop nausea. Ropinirole (Requip®) has been FDA approved for treatment of RLS in adults, but its long-term effects in children with RLS is unknown. Nevertheless, the use of dopaminergic medications may be considered in children with severe cases of RLS, such as described in the case study of Sam G. Opioids should be avoided because of their respiratory depressant effects and potential for dependence.

In the case of secondary RLS due to iron deficiency, there are no existing guidelines for the treatment of children. Iron levels should not be measured when the child is ill, because levels increase during illness. Iron supplementation for children with RLS and low ferritin should be implemented and monitored by a pediatrician or sleep specialist. Once the child's ferritin level is within the normal range, the pediatrician or sleep specialist may recommend a multivitamin containing iron for maintaining iron stores. As in adults, iron supplementation for secondary RLS symptoms in children can take weeks to months to become effective.

COPING STRATEGIES*

In addition to appropriate medication, parents and the entire family must address the child or adolescent's psychological and physical health in dealing with RLS. This section explores the manner in which parents and children can develop coping strategies to deal with the impact of a childhood diagnosis of RLS. It details how parents, in a proactive manner, can develop coping strategies within the family unit. In addition, this section presents specific coping mechanisms that individual children and adolescents can use to minimize the effects of RLS. These mechanisms focus on behavioral issues that can accentuate or alleviate RLS symptoms. It also addresses how parents can help children while they are in the classroom.

---

*The remainder of this chapter was contributed by Karla M. Dzienkowski, RN, BSN, who is the mother of a child with RLS.

A confirmed diagnosis of RLS can serve as a basis for a request for accommodations in the educational setting. Working together, parents and children need to develop a set of positive coping strategies to deal with this potentially long-term health condition, because coping strategies can significantly enhance the child's quality of life.

The Coping Process and the Role of Parents

Coping is a human response to perceived or actual stress. Our personality characteristics, past experiences, and situational views determine our response to an emotionally challenging situation. The parents are at ground zero in the coping process. The coping mechanisms they implement will directly affect all of the family members and how well they adapt to the challenges of having a family member with RLS. The majority of parents develop healthy coping mechanisms that benefit the emotional, social, and medical needs of the affected child and the rest of the family. The effectiveness of the parents' coping skills is directly associated with lower levels of anxiety and depressive feelings in children who have RLS.

The parents and extended family must become proactive in developing coping strategies, because RLS can have an effect on the emotional, social, and intellectual development of the child. Effective coping measures also serve as a foundation as the child matures into adulthood and gains control of their RLS. Parents should become knowledgeable about RLS as well as their child's specific medical diagnosis. The RLS Foundation pamphlet *Restless Legs Syndrome and Periodic Limb Movement Disorder in Children and Adolescents* is a comprehensive and detailed source of information for parents and health care providers (www.rls.org).

The Child's Ability to Cope with RLS

A child recently diagnosed with RLS will experience a variety of emotions. These feelings can vary depending upon age, gender, personality, and emotional maturity. It is not uncommon for the child to feel angry, sad, or to wonder why their body is not working as it should. Some children feel relieved when they are diagnosed because the symptoms they have been experiencing are validated and treatment can begin. Children will vary as to whether they fully share their emotions and feelings with their parents, friends, and family. Some children may be extremely open; others may internalize their feelings. Open lines of communication between the parents and the child with RLS are essential. A warm, caring, and accepting atmosphere will enable the child to feel comfortable with sharing feelings and specific concerns, so a coping strategy can be developed. Some children may not be able to verbalize their feelings and emotions, and information about the child's ability to cope may need to come from observing the child's actions.

> Open lines of communication between
> parents and the child with RLS are essential.

Children with RLS must deal not only with physical issues, but with social and emotional issues as well. Children with RLS may experience (1) a lack of interest in school and/or friends, (2) changes in eating and sleep patterns, (3) generalized sadness, (4) a decrease in academic performance, or (5) other changes in their normal living patterns. The relationship between anxiety disorders and depression is a well-documented finding in adults with RLS (see Chapter 10). Thus, medical management of RLS in children should include the evaluation and treatment of anxiety and depressive feelings. Regardless of the cause of depressive symptoms, parents need to be aware of this possibility and address the situation in a proactive manner. If necessary, talking with a therapist individually or as a family may be beneficial.

Coping Strategies for Adolescents

Adolescence is a pivotal time in life when the formation of self-identity occurs and personality, values, beliefs, self-image, and career choices are made. Teenagers need the support of family, friends, and teachers to help make these choices based on the realistic expectations of living with a chronic condition such as RLS. For a teen, balancing home life, school, and a long-term health condition can be a challenge. It is not uncommon for teens with RLS to have feelings of wanting to live a "normal" life—free from dealing with medication schedules, dietary restrictions, and sleep requirements. Teens want and need to start developing autonomy and confidence, which includes managing their own health care. Most importantly, adolescents who are responsible for their own care are likely to follow the prescribed treatment routine. Parents can remind their teenagers with RLS of the following ways to cope:

1. *Like yourself and your body:* You are a special and unique person. Everyone has limitations, not just people with health concerns.
2. *Hobbies and special abilities:* Everyone is good at something. Explore and find out what you like and find pleasure in doing. For example, take an art class, learn to play an instrument, or become a community volunteer. Developing a hobby or activity that you enjoy helps to build confidence.
3. *Friends and activities:* Build a network of support. Keep up with friends. Join a club at school or in the community.
4. *Be active in your health care:* Do not be shy! Ask your doctor about any concerns you have. By working together, you may learn some strategies to cope with your symptoms. In addition, by communicating directly with your doctor, you will be able to get the treatment that is best suited to your needs.
5. *Physical activity:* Moderate exercise is a great way to relieve stress, feel good, improve sleep, and keep in shape.
6. *Journals:* Journaling is a great outlet to express your thoughts, feelings, and concerns.

The Role of the Family in Developing Coping Strategies

RLS can have minimal impact on family life, or it can have a significant impact. Balancing the needs of a child with RLS with that of the other family members can be challenging. Developing a set of coping strategies can help in the overall adjustment of the affected child and family. Dealing with RLS openly at home and with extended family, friends, and teachers is the best approach for coping with RLS. Listed below are several steps that can help families and children take charge of RLS. These recommendations are a starting point; you may even have a few of your own to add to the list. Obviously, these steps must be tailored to the age and developmental level of the child and the particular details of the RLS condition.

Steps for Coping

1. *Recognize and acknowledge feelings:* Having a support network of friends and family is an important resource for emotional support. Although they may not have an answer (or RLS), they can be great listeners when needed. Join a support group.

2. *Play an active role in your health care:* Knowledge is power. Read and learn all that you can. Prepare a list of questions to ask your doctor before your child's visit so you can have them answered. Your physician's nurse is another excellent source of information. If your pediatrician is not the physician who is treating your child's RLS, be sure to keep him up to date on any changes in your child's care, such as a new medication or dosage changes.

3. *Lifestyle:* Lifestyle changes are part of coping with a chronic condition. Learn the child's RLS triggers and help the child avoid them. In time, these accommodations will become part of the child's daily routine.

4. *Self-advocacy:* Educating and explaining your child's health condition to others is important. Family and friends may be afraid to ask questions, but they still want to know how to help. Know your child's medications and potential side effects. Ask your physician or pharmacist if you have questions about your child's medications. Each parent and the child with RLS should carry an RLS Medical Alert Card to avoid the administration of medication that can cause problems. Give the RLS Medical Alert Card to all of your physicians so they can use it as a point of reference. Parents should also provide a card to the school nurse's office so it is on file in case a medical situation arises. It is a good idea to laminate the card for children (most copy stores provide lamination services for a nominal fee). The Appendix of this book

gives information on how to obtain these cards. A medic alert bracelet or necklace is also a good option for children in case of emergency.

5. *Build on your strengths:* Encourage and help your child find activities he or she enjoys. It will boost his or her self-esteem and serve as an emotional outlet.

6. *Feed your emotional health:* Keep your spirits high. RLS can wreak havoc on your emotions. Watch for signs of depression. Rely on family and friends for support. Let your doctor know if you or your child has any concerns about depression or anxiety.

7. *Sense of humor:* Humor is the best medicine! Just the name RLS usually gets some interesting responses from others.

Helping Siblings Cope

Being the sibling of a child with RLS can be difficult. Open and honest lines of communication are important to help siblings understand the implications of a long-term health condition in a brother or sister. It is not uncommon for them to feel confused or worried about their own health and the health of their sibling. Sometimes, they must take on added responsibilities or assume the role of the older sibling, even though they are younger. At other times, parents are viewed as giving the sibling with RLS preferential treatment. It may be difficult at times to understand why a change in plans has to be made. Teach your child with RLS, and any other children in the family, these important values: being nonjudgmental of others who have difficulties, empathy, allegiance to family, and maturity at an early age.

Parents may need to devote a disproportionate amount of time to the child who has RLS. The actual or perceived difference in time spent with the child with RLS will be noticed by the other family members. Parents must be aware of how the other children are handling the situation. It is best to let them share their feelings and be truthful about what is going on. Many children may be sympathetic for a short period of time, after which they develop resentment towards their parents or the sibling with RLS. Parents need to spend quality time with all of their children, individually. An effective way to accomplish balance is to nurture different interests in each child. Balance and flexibility are critical for a family living with a chronic condition such as RLS.

Management of Care

Parents should include the child in the treatment of his or her RLS. For younger children, use age-appropriate language to help them to learn and understand their treatment plan. Knowledge is an important tool that every child needs to feel more in control. They will be more willing to follow the recommended treatment plan if they are involved in its development. They know their bodies best and should be included in treatment decisions. As children mature, they learn to self-manage their RLS and may want to take a greater role in their life and health care. Parents need to foster this independence because it is an expected part of normal growth and development. The parent takes on the role of "supervisor of care," and the child takes on the role as the daily "manager of care." As supervisor, you still need to watch over the child's management style. This approach is essential, because parents cannot be expected to be present in every situation where a good decision needs to be made. In this way, children will be able to learn the importance of becoming their own advocate.

Noncompliance Issues

One of the difficult issues that a parent of a child with a long-term illness faces is the child's noncompliance with the treatment program. The first instinct is to take over and manage the child's care. This appears to be a great solution: Give them advice and make sure they follow it. However, ownership of the problem belongs to the child or adolescent. Part of growing up and learning to be responsible includes making mistakes, such as skipping or forgetting a medication dose, eating a forbidden food, or staying up too late. This is especially true when teens begin to assert their independence.

Children and adolescents, like adults, need to feel in control of their illness and treatment. When problems arise, be open and use your listening skills to find out what went wrong and help them to get back on track—it may be due to a lack of knowledge, miscommunication, or lack of problem-solving skills. A recent study found that children and ado-

> Children and adolescents, like adults, need to feel in control of their illness and treatment.

lescents differ in their views, in comparison to adults, as to the cause, treatments, and coping strategies needed to deal with RLS.

Sleep Hygiene

Establishing good sleeping habits at an early age will significantly reduce RLS symptoms and improve daytime functioning in the child with RLS.

Sleepovers

Spending the night with a friend is an exciting event for children and adolescents, and sleepovers are possible, even with RLS. Open communication with the child's friends and their parents will help to alleviate any concerns or questions as to the need for dietary limitations and medication needs. Setting an agreed-upon bedtime will help when younger children are involved. In adolescents, a supportive and understanding friendship group is important, and they will help the child with RLS feel comfortable in making the decision to retire early. As a matter of safety, all medications should be placed in properly labeled childproof containers and kept out of the reach of young children, whether at home or away.

Travel

Having RLS should not get in the way of having fun. Planning ahead will help prevent problems. If you are going to be away from home, it would be best to carry a clearly labeled prescription bottle with a childproof lid so that you can have medication on hand if needed. When traveling, carry all necessary medication in your carry-on bag.

Educating Teachers About RLS

Going to school presents unique challenges for the child or adolescent with RLS. Many school personnel have never heard of this condition and do not have experience in dealing with the needs of a student with RLS in the school environment. Educating the child's teachers and counselors is necessary to ensure a successful school experience. Listed below are several ideas that will help in preparation for meeting with school officials:

1. Notify the school in writing of your child's RLS diagnosis and any secondary diagnosis as soon as possible.

2. Request a meeting with all of the teachers and counselors who will have contact with your child. A counselor can arrange a group meeting with all of the teachers so you do not have to meet with them individually.

3. Prepare for the meeting. Give each teacher, counselor, and the nurse an information packet to read prior to the meeting that contains the following:

    •   A letter describing your child's diagnosis and any special needs. Include your contact information: phone numbers (home, work, and cell) and e-mail address. Ask them to contact you at any time if they have any observations or concerns to share.

    •   The *RLS and Periodic Limb Movement Disorder in Children and Adolescents* pamphlet is a great resource for learning about RLS (www.rls.org). Give a copy to every person your child will come into contact with at school.

    •   A letter from the child's physician stating the diagnosis and any accommodations that may be necessary.

    •   Classroom accommodations and scheduling concerns that you or your child may have. Medication administration instructions, if needed during school hours.

4. Develop an education plan to meet your child's specific needs, including the following:

- Who will serve as a contact person for you to communicate with in the school system? Both the parent and child need an advocate at school. This is why it is important that all school personal in contact with your child receive your letter and invitation to a school meeting. Remember, you are building a support network.
- Parents can ask the teachers to contact the parents if they see a change in the child's usual behavior or other problems that may be related to RLS.
- Classroom accommodations.
- Scheduling needs.
- Testing needs.

5. Periodically reevaluate and modify the education plan, if needed. Listed below are a few scheduling arrangements that might be helpful:

- *Physical education:* Schedule physical education for midday. It is a great opportunity to get rid of some of the excess energy in the child's legs.
- *Front-loaded course schedule:* Have the most difficult courses scheduled in the morning rather than in the afternoon, as they may be better able to focus.
- *First period:* Choose a course that allows easy make-up of missed material. If they have had a bad night and need a little extra sleep, they can do so without getting behind in a major course. Do not abuse this privilege, and check with the teacher to get approval.

Section 504 and RLS

Congress has enacted Section 504 of the Rehabilitation Act, which requires public educational institutions to offer accommodation to children with a disability that substantially impairs one of life's basic functions. In the case of education, it is the ability to learn. Therefore, if a child has a severe case of RLS or RLS combined with another disorder, parents can request that the school offer Section 504 accommodation to the child.

The child may qualify for Section 504 status if their RLS affects their school performance, which would require that the school tailor the educational program to address the needs of the child within the public school system (www.504idea.org). School accommodations may involve scheduling, delayed starts, and other modifications of the curriculum. For example, a child may have limited opportunity to reschedule an examination if the school absence is due to the RLS condition. A child with RLS discomfort during the day may be permitted to stand or leave class at the onset of symptoms. Obviously, if a child has RLS and/or another disorder, the accommodations may include physical, instructional, and behavioral accommodations.

Finding a Physician

Finding a physician who is familiar with RLS in children can be challenging. The pediatric diagnostic criteria are relatively new, and many physicians are not familiar with RLS. It may take more than one office visit to determine the best treatment therapy; therefore, it is important to find a physician who is willing to develop a rapport and work with you as a team in securing the best possible treatment.

A recent study found that adolescents identified trust and listening skills as the two most important features they wanted in a physician. These two relationship criteria need to be taken into account when selecting a physician to manage the care of an adolescent, because it will directly affects the adolescent's willingness to comply with his or her treatment program.

CONCLUSION

RLS is a lifelong condition that has only recently begun to be recognized as having its roots in childhood. The manner in which a child or adolescent copes with RLS is a reflection of the way the parents and family have taken on the challenge of living with RLS. Apart from the necessary medical care, families must focus on how they can best cope with RLS symptoms in day-to-day life. Coping plays an important role in alleviating the effects of RLS on a child's life. Therefore, parents need to develop a coping strategy that includes an open line of communication between all family members. The family approach is critical in helping the child with RLS learn the skills necessary to deal with symptoms. Development of positive coping strategies is an important step for children and adolescents so that they can develop a healthy outlook and feel confident in their ability to be responsible for their RLS treatment as they mature into adulthood.

CHAPTER 12

The Patient's Role in Managing Restless Legs Syndrome

PEOPLE WITH RLS should take a role in managing their illness. This chapter discusses the various ways in which you can take an active approach in managing your symptoms so your RLS will be manageable and you will require less or possibly even no medication. Taking an active role requires effort, but the rewards make it definitely worthwhile.

It is essential that any RLS patient with significant symptoms work in close collaboration with his or her physician, because most physicians are not knowledgeable about RLS and need patient feedback and suggestions. Even experienced RLS specialists can only fine-tune the patient's treatment by working as a team *with* the patient. Treatment success will be limited if the physician and patient are not willing to work together. RLS is a chronic and often progressive disorder with no known cure, but that does not mean you should give up and let the disease rule your life.

People with mild RLS may have to make only minor adjustments in their lifestyle, which often become a part of their daily routine. Many of them may not even realize that the disorder has affected their lives. They may only be reminded of their RLS when they make a significant error, such as taking an antihistamine or going to a movie late in the evening without prior medication. People with moderate to severe RLS must be more aware and vigilant, because even minor transgressions can result in a dramatic increase in symptoms. These situations can be avoided with proper care and planning. This chapter discusses techniques for preventing exacerbations of RLS and managing them when they occur.

> With proper care, most RLS patients can live
> full lives with minimal or no discomfort from
> their RLS symptoms.

The coping strategies outlined in this chapter are suitable for anyone with RLS, but you should select the ones that are appropriate for you. If one method does not help, try different strategies until you succeed.

KNOWLEDGE IS CONTROL

Educating yourself about your condition is essential for all people with RLS. The more you learn about RLS, the more you can prevent exacerbating your symptoms and learn how to control them. This book is a comprehensive source of general information about RLS, and other books and pamphlets on general and specific RLS-related topics are listed in the Appendix. Also listed are useful Web sites. One such site, PubMed (www.ncbi.nlm.nih.gov), permits free literature searches and provides abstracts. They charge a fee to obtain complete articles, and some articles may have to be purchased directly from the journal or publisher.

Talking with other people who have RLS is often one of the most helpful resources. They can share their experiences, offering you new solutions and perspectives on how to handle your own problems. Find a support group in your area and attend the next meeting. For those of you who do not have a support group nearby, there are cyberspace support groups, discussion boards, and forums and chat rooms on the Internet. Get involved with others, and share your experiences and thoughts about RLS.

Join the RLS Foundation. This nonprofit organization raises money for research and education and is also one of the best sources of information on RLS. Their quarterly newsletter, *NightWalkers*, contains the latest information from scientific articles, answers to RLS questions by experts, patient experiences, a column on complementary and alternative medicine, and lots of other interesting information.

It is important to be aware of the medications that tend to *worsen* RLS, and people with RLS, including children, are encouraged to carry a Medical Alert Card containing this information. There cards are par-

> Join a RLS support group and the RLS Foundation.

ticularly helpful when traveling or visiting an emergency room or when seeing a physician who is not familiar with you or RLS. The Appendix of this book gives information on how to obtain these cards.

LIFESTYLE AND DAILY ACTIVITIES

The following suggested lifestyle changes may be minor or quite significant, depending on the severity of your RLS. Most of these adjustments are easy to integrate into your life and often become routine.

Scheduling Activities

As discussed previously, RLS symptoms follow a circadian (24-hour) rhythm. Symptoms are worse in the evening and at night—and better in the morning and early afternoon. Most people are symptom-free in the morning and afternoon, so this is the best time to schedule sedentary activities that tend to aggravate RLS. Morning or early afternoon is the preferred time to go to the movies, read a book, schedule meetings that require sitting, or attend religious services. When scheduling travel, book an early morning trip and avoid evening departures. Many people with RLS report that doing housework is easier in the evening, preferring to leave the more sedentary tasks for the morning.

Some people take advantage of the fluctuation in RLS symptoms by being active until 3–5 A.M. and going to sleep when their RLS symptoms are naturally decreasing; however, people who work may only have a few hours to sleep in order to get to their job. Going to sleep later at night will work better for people who have flexible morning hours and can sleep longer. For others, delaying bedtime may result in sleep deprivation, which may further worsen their RLS. Proper sleep hygiene is important for people with RLS, and you should try to get adequate sleep by observing regular sleep and wake times.

Some women are affected by hormonal changes. They may experience marked worsening of RLS symptoms starting about 1 week before the beginning of their menstrual cycle. Women with hormonal RLS fluctuations should not schedule sedentary activities during this time and should consider an increase in their RLS medications if they are required to be sedentary.

Seasonal changes can also affect people with RLS. Some notice that their symptoms are worse in the summer; others find that winter is worse. Once you determine the time of the year that is difficult for you, try not to schedule vacations that require prolonged airplane or car travel during that time. Schedule sedentary vacations and travel for the time of year when you have the least risk of problems with RLS.

The Bedroom

Sleep deprivation is a constant problem for many people with RLS, because both RLS symptoms and PLMS can disturb sleep. It is important to make the bedroom as conducive as possible for falling asleep. The room should be quiet—if not, consider buying a white noise generator. You can purchase a durable, compact, yet inexpensive white noise generator called the SoundScreen™ on the Internet or at specialty stores.

Controlling the temperature is also important for many people with RLS. Most people sleep better in a cool (but not too cold) environment, and this seems to be the case for many people with RLS. Some people find that their symptoms are worse if the bed covers touch their legs, and so they have frames built to tent the covers away from them. Others need constant pressure, such as elastic stockings, on their legs in order to sleep.

Find an alternative place to sleep if sleeping in your bedroom becomes a problem. You may be so worried about bothering your bed partner that sleep becomes difficult. The temperature may not suit you—although it may suit your bed partner—or the bedroom may be too noisy, especially with a snoring bed partner. Get out of your bedroom when these situations occur, and try sleeping in a more comfortable place; alternatively, your noisy bed partner may leave. Ideally, you should sleep in your own bedroom, although it is not always possible.

People with RLS may need an additional place to sleep for other reasons. Some people find that they need their legs raised, and so they sleep with their feet propped up on the back of the couch. Others find that sleeping on the floor with their feet propped up against a wall reduces RLS symptoms. Figure 12-1 demonstrates one extreme measure taken by a woman with RLS to relieve her symptoms enough to sleep.

Control Your Environment

You may not be able to sit for long periods while performing your daily tasks if you have moderate to severe RLS. You may have to interrupt

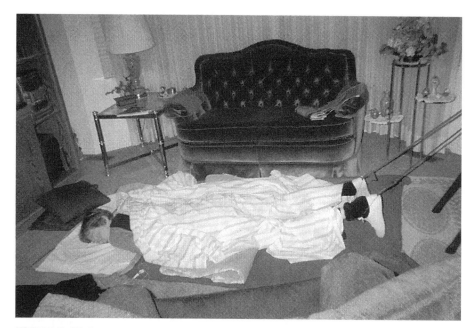

FIGURE 12-1

A RLS patient finds relief by sleeping on the floor with socks and athletic shoes on her feet while a pulley system applies constant tension to her legs.

these tasks frequently to get up and move. However, there are ways to work around this problem. For example, increase your computer or desk height to counter level, with a matching tall stool or chair, so you can continue working while standing. Similarly, keep a bookstand on a high counter or desk for use when you must pace and still wish to read.

A great example of how to control your environment is Pickett Guthrie's (one of the co-founders of the RLS Foundation) solution to avoiding RLS while going on long road trips. Her severe RLS limited her ability to remain sedentary, yet she and her husband Bob were avid travelers. Bob Guthrie devised an ingenious solution to their dilemma. He bought a minivan with three rows of seats, took out the second row, and installed an exercise bicycle so she could peddle away her RLS symptoms while he drove. For more information on this bicycle solution, read Bob Guthrie's letter to Virginia Wilson in her book, *Sleep Thief* (see the Appendix).

Similarly, people who want to watch television or read when bothered by RLS can do so while riding an exercise bicycle at home. This has the added benefit of increasing cardiovascular health. Look at other situations that are limited because of RLS—you may be able to devise new methods of dealing with them.

Temperature seems to affect many people with RLS. Hot, humid weather can exacerbate RLS symptoms. Plan ways to control your environment if hot or cold temperatures affect you. People who are affected by heat can stay indoors with the air-conditioner turned on during this type of weather. Choose places and times of the year to vacation that will not exacerbate your RLS.

When traveling, choose situations that will permit you to walk, when necessary. Make sure you get an aisle seat on airplanes. Do not get trapped into sitting by the window! You can get a note from your physician stating that you must sit in an aisle seat. Better yet, get that physician's note to include sitting in a bulkhead seat with plenty of room to move or even kick your legs without disturbing other passengers. If there is a choice, travel by train rather than bus or car so that you will have ample room to walk and move. When traveling by car, plan frequent stops so you can get out and walk.

Take an aisle seat in the back or near an exit when you go to a movie or concert so you can get up and walk, if necessary. Choose seats that have plenty of legroom. This also applies to other group settings, such as

> Always plan an escape route!

religious services, lectures, and business meetings. Choose mornings for these activities when possible. Take your medication 1–3 hours before the start of the activity. Wear comfortable clothing and bring food, such as popcorn, candy, or raisins, as a distraction. *Always* plan an escape route for any sedentary activity so you will not be physically trapped with your RLS symptoms.

Driving a Motor Vehicle and Car Travel

Although most people with RLS manage to get adequate sleep, many are chronically sleep deprived. This can cause dangerous problems with driving. Lapses of attention or actually falling asleep at the wheel should alert you that RLS has impaired your ability to drive. Daytime sleepiness is one of the most common causes of motor vehicle accidents, and sooner or later you will harm yourself or someone else if you drive when you are sleepy. Many states consider a sleepy driver to be impaired, similar to driving while intoxicated, and may impose fines and even jail sentences. With proper treatment of RLS and insomnia, however, most people with RLS should be able to drive.

Some people with RLS may still be impaired, even when treatment eliminates their symptoms, because some of the RLS medications can cause *increased* sleepiness. These include the dopamine agonists (Table 5-4), anticonvulsants (Table 6-1), long-acting benzodiazepines (Table 5-1), and painkillers (Table 5-3). The dopamine agonists generally cause sleepiness only at higher doses, but some people are more susceptible to this adverse effect. Anticonvulsants typically produce sleepiness as an unwanted side effect. When taken at bedtime, this may actually be a benefit, not a problem. However, the higher bedtime doses that are frequently necessary can cause next-day sleepiness or hangover effects. The longer-acting benzodiazepines often produce sleepiness during the following day. Some people experience sleepiness with daytime use of painkillers. Caution should be taken when using these medications and driving. Whenever starting or increasing the dosage of these drugs, do not drive until you are certain that you are not impaired.

People with RLS may also have PLM while sitting for prolonged periods, and a leg jerk might accidentally hit the brake or gas pedal, causing an unintended change in speed. People who experience this problem should consider medication that decreases these movements.

Some people with RLS find that driving is *easier* than being a passenger, because the level of concentration necessary to drive lessens their RLS symptoms. Others find that driving does not help their RLS and prefer the passenger seat so they can move or stretch their legs at will. Bring your bag of RLS tricks (video games, leg massagers, comfortable pillows, etc.) to help control any unwanted RLS symptoms when you are a passenger on a long road trip.

Managing RLS in the Work Environment

Working is essential for most people with RLS, but problems with concentrating are common, especially when RLS disturbs sleep. The insomnia and RLS should be adequately treated; however, watch for any daytime sleepiness from your RLS medications. Long meetings, deskwork, or other prolonged sedentary activities that worsen RLS are another challenge. Arrange sedentary activities for the morning hours if your work schedule is flexible.

Clearly, some jobs are not appropriate for people with RLS. Shift work is particularly difficult. Changing sleep times may further worsen insomnia and increase daytime sleepiness. Sedentary employment may not be suitable for many people with RLS. However, if you can work with a tall stool and elevated desk or counter or stand while working, you may be able to cope with a sedentary job. To prevent RLS while working at a desk job, rhythmic exercises such as using a Cush Push™ (see Physical Activities, pages 172–173) may be helpful.

If problems with employment occur, it is important for you to discuss them with your supervisors and coworkers in a nonconfrontational manner. Reasonable supervisors and coworkers should be willing to help you with workplace accommodations, although some may not. They may consider you less productive and cause problems. You may need to present written documentation from your physician when you discuss these issues with them. This should protect you if they decide to terminate your employment.

If your job requires you to be sedentary for long hours without the flexibility of changing position, consider finding another job that is more RLS friendly. If you cannot manage your RLS adequately enough to work or cannot find another job, filing for disability is a reasonable option. Information about applying for Social Security disability is provided in Chapter 14.

Some people with RLS find that being self-employed is the best solution. This provides flexibility and control of your work environment. Plus it is easy to avoid the stress and fear of working for a supervisor who may not be supportive.

Avoid Alcohol, Tobacco, and Caffeine

Unfortunately, knowing the importance of avoiding alcohol, tobacco, and caffeine does not always mean that people with RLS will stop using them. These three drugs are addictive when used on a regular basis, and they cause withdrawal symptoms when you stop using them. Not all people with RLS react negatively, but those who do are often unaware that these drugs exacerbate the symptoms of RLS, especially if they used them before they developed RLS.

Zyban® may be a good choice for people with RLS who are smokers and want to quit. This is the same drug (bupropion) as the RLS-friendly antidepressant Wellbutrin®. Zyban® has been shown to significantly reduce the desire to smoke and should not increase the symptoms of RLS.

People with RLS who love to drink coffee might feel better if they restrict their consumption to one or two cups in the morning. Coffee later in the day is more likely to provoke RLS symptoms. There are many other caffeinated beverages that should be avoided. Tea and colas are obvious sources of caffeine, but many soft drinks, even clear-colored ones, contain significant amounts of caffeine. Additionally, many foods and drugs contain caffeine and should be avoided, if possible. People with RLS should become familiar with the numerous products that contain caffeine. See the following Web site for a list of the foods containing caffeine and in what amounts: http://www.cspinet.org/new/cafchart.htm.

Alcohol often presents a problem because most social drinkers prefer their alcoholic beverages in the evening. On the evenings when alcohol is consumed, people with RLS should be prepared to suffer from increased symptoms or prevent them by taking extra RLS medication beforehand. With a little planning, most people with RLS should be able to tolerate a few alcoholic drinks on occasion.

Dietary Issues

As discussed in Chapter 4, there is no scientific information available on the effect of nutrition in RLS. However, many people with RLS have noticed that certain foods or groups of foods affect them adversely. It may be helpful to keep a dietary log and a sleep diary (available at www.rls.org) to see which foods, if any, are triggers for your RLS. Avoiding foods and beverages containing caffeine and alcohol should be considered as part of these dietary changes.

Exercise

Mild to moderate levels of regular exercise are usually quite beneficial for people with RLS. Excessive exercise tends to aggravate RLS, especially when the RLS is severe. The best time of day to exercise can vary considerably. Some people prefer exercising early in the day; for others, the beneficial effects may only last a few hours, so they exercise in the evening to help relieve symptoms before bedtime. However, exercising too vigorously too close to bedtime can cause increased arousals, which can prevent restful sleep. Only trial and error can determine the most appropriate exercise habits for any individual. Many people prefer aerobic exercises such as walking, running, or bicycling. Others prefer yoga, Pilates, or other stretching techniques. Experiment with several forms of exercise until you determine the routine that works best to control your RLS symptoms.

FIND YOUR RLS TRIGGERS AND AVOID THEM

People with RLS often do things that worsen their symptoms, but they are unaware of it. Medications, diet, and daily activities may bother some people with RLS. Just because a drug or other trigger is listed as being "RLS unfriendly" does not mean that it will aggravate *your* RLS. Some of these triggers may even help your RLS. Before you can avoid triggers, you must first determine which of the potential problems actually affect you.

Food Triggers

The best way to find your triggers is to divide the potential triggers into manageable groups and tackle them one at a time; for example, start with dietary triggers. Do not make any drastic changes at once. Try changing only one item at a time and see how it affects you. To determine the effect of carbohydrates on your RLS, you may first decide to eliminate simple carbohydrates such as sugar. Give the change a week or two before making up your mind because RLS fluctuates from day to day. After testing simple carbohydrates, complex carbohydrates, such as bread and rice, can be examined. Another option would be to eliminate only gluten-containing complex carbohydrates (wheat) and see if you experience an improvement in your condition.

It can be time-consuming and tedious to go through the dietary changes one at a time. However, this is the only way you can be sure that changing your diet is really helping. Keep a log and sleep diary to document how potential triggers affect you. By using this systematic approach, you should be able to determine your own personal RLS triggers. Test different foods in the same way as carbohydrates. Many people with RLS find that eating ice cream aggravates their symptoms. Be sure to evaluate foods containing caffeine.

Medication Triggers

The medications that worsen RLS should be carefully evaluated. If you taking an RLS-unfriendly drug that is important for treating another problem, be careful when attempting to see if it affects your RLS. Stopping a necessary drug can be dangerous. Before using trial and error to test whether a drug is worsening your RLS, discuss the situation with your physician. If the drug is affecting your RLS, your physician can change it to one that does not.

Clothing Triggers

Many people with RLS find that tight-fitting clothes worsen their symptoms. Others find that certain materials are especially bothersome. Experiment with different clothing to find out what works best for you.

Activities, Including Time, Duration, and Level

Any sedentary activity can trigger RLS, but you should determine how early in the day the activity will bring on symptoms; for example, watching television at 9:00 P.M. may be a problem, but not at 7:00 P.M. Record shows that come on late and watch them at a more RLS-friendly time. The duration of sedentary activities is also important. You may be able to sit for hours in the morning, but only for a few minutes in the late evening. Determine how long you can sit still at any time of the day and plan accordingly. When you take a long car trip, leave early in the morning and stop more frequently as the day progresses.

Daytime activities that fatigue your legs or body, in general, will often provoke RLS in the evening. Walking excessively has a high potential of exacerbating RLS. Determine the level of activity that you can tolerate and limit it accordingly. If possible, spread the more arduous activities out over several days.

Stress

Situations that trap you—by denying you an easy escape route to move and walk around—will more predictably aggravate RLS. Avoid these situations as much as possible, because they can worsen symptoms beyond your ability to control them. Proper planning should eliminate most of these situations, but stress can be difficult to avoid, and you may have to deal with it occasionally.

FIND YOUR RLS RELIEVERS AND USE THEM

People with RLS should develop a list of everything that lessens their RLS symptoms. This includes medication and nondrug treatments. Jill Gunzel, also known as "the RLS Rebel," calls this "gathering your bag of tricks." It is important to have your bag of tricks available and ready to use at any time because you cannot always be sure when RLS symptoms will occur. Jill's Web site (http://rlsrebel.com) has an excellent description on how to "pack your bag" with these tricks and a comprehensive approach to using them that she calls the B.O.T.A. (Bag of Tricks Approach). Jill also discusses numerous tricks that help relieve RLS symptoms and the situations for which they are best suited. Review Jill's Web site for its wealth of RLS information and unique approach to managing and coping with RLS. Jill is also the author of *Restless Legs Syndrome: The RLS Rebel's Survival Guide* (see Appendix).

Identifying the "tricks" that will relieve your RLS symptoms requires trial and error. Some of the tricks that help others will not help you, but you should certainly try them. Develop as large a bag of tricks as possible, because some of them work well in certain situations, but not in others. Playing a computer or video game will help get you through a long plane flight, but is clearly not suitable for fending off RLS symptoms during a movie or religious service.

People who require daily preventative therapy with a dopamine agonist or gabapentin for their RLS often need additional types of medication for particular situations or unanticipated symptoms. The dopamine agonists are effective when taken 1–2 hours before RLS symptoms occur, but they are not too helpful when RLS is active. Once symptoms begin, levodopa, a narcotic, or a sleeping pill (if it is time to go to sleep) work more quickly and are thus more appropriate. At times, situations arise in which there is insufficient time to take preventive medications, or patients simply forget to take their medication. Additionally, there will be times when the standard dose of a preventive medication does not work as well and the patient needs a quick fix for his or her RLS symptoms. Even people with well-controlled RLS should have quick-acting medications available for those times when relief is needed. The following techniques for controlling RLS are essential for those times when your medication does not work, is not appropriate, or is not available.

1. Mental Activities
    - Video or computer games
    - Puzzles (crossword, jigsaw, word, math, or logic)
    - Card games (solitaire, if alone)
    - Knitting
    - Music, with or without headphones, especially if you mentally or physically sing along, tap your foot, or move your body
    - Conversation, especially discussing interesting issues or arguing
    - Homework, balancing a checkbook, paperwork
    - Writing a diary, letter, or Internet blog
2.. Physical Activities
    - *Walking:* This activity is used by RLS patients every day.
    - *Stretching:* With or without aids such as elastic bands, this activity is particularly helpful in sedentary situations. There are many different types and ways to stretch; try to find the ones that work for you. Experiment with them and explore stretches that have helped other people with RLS.
    - *Leg Exercises:* Stretching and any other exercise that works the calf and thigh muscles will be beneficial. Exercises that involve movement at the ankle joint are especially helpful for sedentary activities. The Cush Push™ is a double-chambered, inflatable pillow that is available on the Internet. The inflated cushion is rhythmically "pushed" by your feet. Other pillows often work as

well as the Cush Push™. Many people use foot tapping and leg shaking as RLS relievers when they are unable to get up and walk.

3. Sexual Activities
    *   Sexual activities can relieve RLS symptoms, including sexual intimacy with a partner or masturbation. Occasionally, sexual activities may worsen RLS.

4. Counterstimulation
    *   *Hot or Cold Water:* Baths or showers can be helpful in calming restless legs. Some people alternate hot and/or cold water, run from the faucet directly over their legs. Hot or cold packs may work equally well.
    *   *Leg Massage:* Self-massage or having someone else massage your legs can be very helpful. Self-massage is especially useful in sedentary situations, such as movies, meetings, and airplane travel. Some people prefer electrical massagers.

5. Distractions
    *   *Food and Drink:* Many people with RLS notice that certain foods diminish their symptoms. It is not understood whether this is due to the distraction of the eating process or the food itself. Foods such as pistachios are particularly helpful for some people because consuming them requires more effort. Drinking herbal tea can be calming.
    *   *Reading:* It is quite likely that the benefits of reading interesting magazines or books may be due to mental stimulation, but the distraction value might also be part of the process.
    *   *Aromas:* Incense, scented candles, and other smells may distract you from your RLS symptoms, enabling you to sit for longer periods.

LISTEN TO YOUR BODY AND DO NOT CROSS THE RLS LINE!

People with RLS are often aware of a "line" that should not be crossed—or their symptoms will worsen dramatically. Once this happens, it is usually difficult to get control of these intense RLS symptoms. Many people

> There is no good reason to fight the urge to move.

try to fight their RLS symptoms and end up crossing the line. There is no good reason to fight the urge to move.

Act as early as possible to avoid symptom worsening. Most people can sense when their symptoms are about to start. RLS symptoms are often preceded by an increase in general anxiety or other vague sensations. Listen to your body, and once you know your warning signs, act quickly to prevent crossing the RLS line and getting to the point of no return. The most obvious thing to do is get up and start walking, but you can use anything in your bag of tricks.

Remember, it is always easier to prevent RLS symptoms than treat existing symptoms; however, this usually requires some forethought. If your RLS symptoms tend to start at 10:00 P.M., take preventive measures a few hours earlier. This can include taking your RLS medication, going for a walk, or doing your stretching exercises from 7 to 9 P.M. Use whatever you have in your bag of RLS tricks to ward off symptoms. Combine two or more, and they may work even better. Experiment with the choice and timing of your preventive techniques until you are sure they will consistently prevent the onset of RLS. Remember to act early enough so that you do not ever cross the RLS line and suffer needlessly.

ANGER, FRUSTRATION, DEPRESSION, AND ANXIETY

Anger and Frustration

Living with RLS usually provokes strong emotions. Sleep is often disrupted and daytime activities are limited, and it is easy to be angry and frustrated when others do not understand what you are going through. Frustration and anger can really increase when that lack of understanding includes your physician and prevents you from getting proper care.

You did not choose to have RLS, but you can choose the manner in which you react to living with it. The anger and frustration that come so easily do not lead to anything positive. These emotions can destroy your personal relationships, and they certainly do not help you get better medical care. Try to channel your negative emotions into positive action. Instead of being a victim, fight the disorder, not the other people around you who only want to help. Remember, with current treatment, most people with RLS attain satisfactory control of their symptoms. Channel your energies into educating yourself and others about RLS. This will probably include educating your physician. Everyone will be much more willing to interact with you when you are positive. Consider getting professional counseling if you have difficulty with negative emotions. You can also participate in an RLS support group, where you can learn how to express your feelings and receive support and understanding from others.

Discuss your feelings with your family and close friends, but make sure you have already achieved some control. It may be difficult for people who are close to you to be helpful when your anger and frustration levels are high. However, if you can educate your family, friends, and coworkers, they will be more understanding and helpful when your RLS symptoms make you appear to be acting oddly. Hopefully, you can make them comprehend that RLS is a real disorder and you are not just making up crazy symptoms.

Depression

Studies have found that depression is common in people with RLS and can occur before or after the onset of RLS. It is easy to understand how people with untreated or improperly treated RLS can be depressed. Insomnia and fatigue, which are so common with RLS, are independent risk factors for depression. If the depression occurred after the onset of RLS, treating the RLS can resolve much or all of the depression. When treatment of RLS eliminates insomnia, fatigue, and other symptoms, there is a good chance that it will also eliminate most, if not all of the depression. Patients may even be able to eliminate their antidepressant medications after effective treatment of RLS.

Depression that exists prior to the onset of RLS generally worsens significantly once RLS symptoms manifest. Patients may need several medications to treat their depression; however, most antidepressant medications tend to worsen RLS. Stopping or changing them may be difficult or impossible. Physicians should first treat the RLS symptoms so the level of depression and need for treatment can be assessed.

It may seem obvious that depressed people should know they are depressed; however, this is not always the case. To diagnose depression, a person needs to experience five of the nine diagnostic criteria listed in Table 12-1. You should get medical help as soon as possible if you suspect that you or someone close to you is depressed. Although some physicians who treat RLS may be comfortable treating depression, it may require a psychiatrist or other mental health specialist working in conjunction with the physician who is treating the RLS. Depression is a serious illness that should be managed by well-trained professionals.

Table 12-1 Symptoms of Major Depression
Depressed mood
Diminished interests
Feeling worthless
Thoughts of death
Weight change
Insomnia or hypersomnia (increased sleepiness)
Fatigue or loss of energy
Diminished concentration
Psychomotor retardation or agitation

Anxiety

Anxiety also occurs commonly in people with RLS. The feeling of restlessness in the affected limb often feels like an "anxious" limb, and many people find this extends to a generalized feeling of anxiety. People will frequently have increased anxiety as they anticipate the occurrence of their RLS symptoms, knowing they will not be able to sit, lie down, or fall asleep later in the day. Bedtime is especially feared, because people with RLS often toss and turn, unable to fall asleep, or they walk around the house for hours. As the day progresses, anxiety levels increase in anticipation of entering the bedroom. While being tormented in their bedroom every night, anxiety increases as they ponder how to get through the next sleep-deprived day.

Frequently, anxiety occurs with depression. When this happens, the treatment may be similar to that for depression, because many of the antidepressant medications also help anxiety. When the anxiety component is more severe than the depression, additional medication such as benzodiazepine sedatives may be beneficial. Anxiety occurring without depression is generally treated similarly to when it is combined with depression.

Anxiety creates additional problems for people with RLS because it can heighten the level of RLS symptoms. Furthermore, as anxiety levels increase, approaching panic, it becomes difficult to think logically about what to do to control the worsening symptoms. It is easy for people with RLS who become physically trapped for extended periods of time to panic and lose the ability to help themselves.

To prevent panic and increasing anxiety, people with RLS should include anxiety-relieving techniques in their bag of RLS tricks. These might include meditation, controlled breathing practices, biofeedback methods, muscle and general relaxation techniques, and visualization

> Maintain a large bag of "RLS tricks" and use them to prevent crossing the RLS line and entering into the panic zone.

and self-hypnosis. You can learn anxiety-reducing aids on your own or from a mental health professional. It does take significant time and effort to learn these techniques, and regular practice is required for them to remain effective. By maintaining a large bag of RLS tricks, you should be able to avoid *crossing the RLS line* and entering into the panic zone.

People who are anxious can also benefit from talking to others in similar situations. If support groups and talking with family and friends is not helpful, consider seeing a mental health professional. Anxiety is miserable to live with, and it is important to treat it in order to break the vicious cycle of anxiety increasing RLS, which, in turn, further increases anxiety.

Nocturnal Eating and Weight Gain

It is common for people with moderate to severe RLS to spend a significant part of the night awake and moving, rather than sleeping. Eating is one of the activities that often helps fill the boring nighttime hours. Many "nightwalkers" gain between 30 and 50 pounds as a secondary result of their RLS. This is sometimes the only reason their RLS difficulties come to the attention of their physician. The simplest solution is to treat the nighttime RLS so people can sleep at night. Unfortunately, some people may be difficult to treat or they may be reluctant to take medication.

People who remain awake most nights and are gaining weight should consider other solutions. Food serves as a distraction from their RLS symptoms. Try preparing low-calorie snacks, such as celery and carrot sticks, which can be substituted for high-calorie snacks. Eating low-calorie snacks during the night can help relieve boredom and serve as a distraction without putting on extra pounds.

Medical Situations

Medical situations can be particularly difficult for people with RLS. Surgery is discussed in Chapter 9; other medical situations are discussed below.

Radiology Tests

The radiology tests that present the greatest difficulty for people with RLS include computed tomography (CT) and MRI scans. These tests require you to be immobile from 30 minutes up to 1–2 hours. This is almost impossible for some people with RLS, although many can get through these examinations with proper treatment. People who are properly treated should already know the amount of medication they need for different sedentary situations; however, they may need extra medication for CT and MRI scans. Going into the dark tunnel of the scanner's tube and the forced immobility can provoke marked anxiety, which can worsen RLS. Take dopamine agonists 1–3 hours before the procedure if they help you. Adding a small dose of a painkiller or benzodiazepine may be helpful. The benzodiazepine sedatives are especially beneficial because they decrease anxiety.

If RLS symptoms occur during the scan, despite your best efforts to prevent them, the physician performing the procedure can give you an injection of a narcotic, such as meperidine, which should stop the RLS symptoms quickly. Discuss this potential problem and treatment with the physician prior to the procedure so that he or she will be ready and willing to give you an injection, if necessary. Prepare in advance for these tests, and they will not be so frightening.

Emergency Room Visits

Your regular physician likely knows your health issues, including your RLS; however, when you go to the emergency room (ER), you cannot pick your physician. Unfortunately, most ER physicians know little about RLS. These busy physicians use many drugs that aggravate RLS, and it is quite common to hear horror stories about people with RLS who have their symptoms exacerbated after receiving medication in the ER, often a sedating antihistamine such as diphenhydramine. The best way to guard against this is to learn all you can about the drugs that exacerbate RLS and carry your RLS Medical Alert Card with you at all times. Hopefully, you will never enter the ER in the unconscious state, but it is still be a good idea to have a medical alert bracelet or necklace identifying you as a person with RLS

FINAL MESSAGE: DO NOT GIVE UP UNTIL YOUR RLS IS UNDER CONTROL!

Most people with RLS should be able to control their symptoms. This may not happen with the first drug or physician visit, although it is certainly possible in mild cases. For many people, however, control of symptoms requires considerable effort on the part of the patient and physician. Many different drugs or combinations of drugs might have to be tried. There may be adverse reactions on the road to finding the correct therapeutic regimen for any individual. Remember, there are many different possible treatments, and you and your physician should explore as many of them as it takes to find relief.

A small percentage of people with RLS do not find relief. Some of them cannot tolerate any of the RLS medications, or they are not helped by the ones they can tolerate. One potential problem in these difficult cases may be the incorrect use of medication. The doses of the drugs or combinations used may not be optimal. You may need to find a physician with more experience and expertise in treating RLS (see Chapter 15). With the aid of a knowledgeable, caring physician and the available medical treatments, most people with RLS will find relief from their symptoms. The pace of research is increasing dramatically, and new treatments are being developed and tested. Do not give up until your RLS symptoms are under control!

CHAPTER 13

Applying for Social Security Disability

A PPLYING TO THE SOCIAL SECURITY ADMINISTRATION (SSA) for disability can be a frustrating and tedious task. There are multiple forms to fill out and numerous evaluations to obtain from your physicians. After making your case for disability, you will need to wait for a long period of time (6–12 months) for a seemingly arbitrary decision as to whether you will receive disability. Only 30 percent of disability applications will be approved after the first step of the process. After failing to obtain disability, it is common to find other applicants who are successful despite ostensibly weaker cases. You can always appeal your decision—perseverance and persistence are important for ultimate success.

You will not receive disability based solely on your RLS, even if your disorder is severe. This disorder is not well known, and those granting disability need to know if the problems resulting from your RLS are severe enough to warrant disability. For example, if your RLS is causing insomnia resulting in daytime sleepiness severe enough to prevent you from performing any type of work, you may have a good case.

There are medical tests that can accurately document the level of excessive daytime sleepiness, and they should support your claim powerfully. These tests include an overnight sleep study, which is especially helpful as evidence for disruptive PLMD, an MSLT (Multiple Sleep Latency Test), which consists of four to five monitored daytime nap studies), and a MWT (Maintenance of Wakefulness Test), which consists of four to five monitored sessions of trying to stay awake while resting. Submitting this type of objective documentation to support your disability will help strengthen your claim.

There have been several cases of people with RLS obtaining disability. Success may vary from state to state and depending on who reviews your case. You must follow all the rules, present all the paperwork, and make sure that you have done enough legwork to support your case as strongly as possible. This often includes explaining RLS to the reviewers of your claim. Do not be discouraged if your initial appeal fails; a large fraction of claims are only sustained on appeal. You should be ready to undertake the appeal process in order to maximize your chances of success.

The Job Accommodation Network (http://www.jan.wvu.edu/links/adalinks.htm) has information about work and disability, including many links to the rules and regulations of work and disability. The EEOC (Equal Employment Opportunity Commission, http://www.eeoc.gov/) also has information about work and disability. You can get application forms, additional information, or a referral to the National Organization of Social Security Claimant's Representatives from the SSA.

The following helpful information is taken from an article titled "Social Security Disability and RLS," which was published in the RLS Foundation's quarterly newsletter *NightWalkers* in 2002.

If you are unable to work because of RLS, you may be entitled to receive monthly disability payments under either of two disability programs administered by the Social Security Administration. The first program is Social Security Disability (SSD) insurance, which is based on the taxes you have paid into the system. The second, Supplemental Security Income (SSI), is based on financial need. Severe, uncontrollable RLS can be disabling in itself, or it can be a contributing factor when there are additional impairments that limit your capacity for work. Unfortunately, it is difficult to prove that you have RLS and even more difficult to prove that it prevents you from working. If you apply for disability benefits, you should know how the system works, and you should be prepared to take a proactive approach toward shepherding your claim though the process.

In most states, disability decisions are made at five levels: the initial level, the reconsideration level, the Office of Hearings and Appeals (OHA), the Appeals Council, and the court system. Some cases have been appealed and won in the U.S. Supreme Court. The first two levels (initial and reconsideration) are adjudicated by state agencies called *Disability*

Determination Services (DDS). A new system that streamlines the process and eliminates the reconsideration step is being tested in 10 states.

The SSA disability system is generally fair, but not fast. If you cannot work because of physical or mental medical conditions, you will normally receive benefits—eventually. People who apply for benefits on the basis of RLS are often unsuccessful until they appear before an Administrative Law Judge (ALJ) at the OHA. It may take a year or more to obtain an OHA determination, and attorneys' fees may absorb a large portion of any retroactive award. The trick is to have benefits awarded at an early stage.

There are three basic obstacles to an early favorable outcome on a disability claim based on RLS.

1. *Your description of your symptoms is not enough to qualify you for benefits. You must have a medically determinable impairment.* A disability decision is based on medical evidence. There are no diagnostic tests or a specific set of signs and symptoms that establish a diagnosis of RLS. The diagnosis is typically based on the clinical history taken by a knowledgeable treating physician who is familiar with both RLS and your particular circumstances.

    Your own treating physician is always the preferred source of information. The SSA will attempt to secure this information, but it is frequently either inadequate or unobtainable for various reasons. If SSA cannot obtain sufficient information from existing sources, they will arrange and pay for a disability examination with a consulting physician. In most cases the consulting physician will not be familiar with your circumstances and probably will not find any physical evidence of RLS to support your claim.

2. *Despite advances in recent years, the medical community remains poorly educated concerning the functional effects or even the existence of RLS.* Although a relatively common disorder, RLS remains unknown to many in the medical field. Disability adjudicators, review physicians, and ALJs may not realize what a devastating impact RLS can have on a person's ability to work, and they may not know how to evaluate it appropriately under the complex SSA regulations. You may have to

educate them by including material such as the RLS Foundation's Medical Bulletin with your disability application.

3. The SSA does not have specific criteria for the assessment of RLS, PLMD, or other sleep disorders. The SSA has a *Listing of Impairments*, which consists of a broad spectrum of impairments that are considered *disabling*. If you do not *meet a listing*, you can still qualify if you have an impairment or combination of impairments that impose functional limitations *equivalent* to one of the listed impairments. Unfortunately, there is no listing for RLS or even a listing that is comparable. It is important to furnish SSA with a detailed description of your own particular limitations because it will have to stand on its own merits.

If you do not qualify on the basis of medical considerations alone, SSA uses a complex process that assesses your *functional limitations*. If you cannot resume your usual work activity, SSA will consider your age, education, and relevant work experience to determine if you have *transferable skills* to other forms of work.

The good news is that there is a renewed emphasis on incorporating into the decision-making process the opinions of treating physicians and the testimony of disability applicants themselves. You may shorten the assessment process, improve your chances of a favorable decision, and avoid unnecessary examinations if you obtain a report from your own physician and submit it when you file your application. (Be sure to keep a copy.) A simple statement that you have RLS and are *disabled* is not sufficient. Your physician's report should include a treatment history, relevant clinical observations, test results, dates first and last seen, frequency of visits, and a diagnosis and prognosis, plus a functional assessment of how your problem or problems limit your ability to work.

This functional assessment or *medical source statement* is one of the most important pieces of information in any disability case. The SSA is less concerned with the nature of your impairment than they are with how it affects your ability to function. Your treating physician's opinion concerning what work-related activities you can no longer perform will serve as the *controlling factor* in the decision-making process unless there is clear evidence that refutes it.

Functional assessments are generally expressed as quantified estimates of how long or how much you can sit, stand, walk, lift, carry, bend, stoop, climb, etc. Other work-related limitations that may be associated with RLS include daytime fatigue, drowsiness and lack of energy, and impaired ability to concentrate, remember instructions, stay within a schedule, maintain attendance, arrive at work on time, or keep up an acceptable pace. Your physician's report should include an appraisal of such factors when relevant.

Some RLS medications can be potent. The report should address any significant physical or mental side effects that you may be experiencing from drugs or any other therapy. If you have secondary depression or anxiety, an assessment of how these problems further impact your ability to work is important. It would be worth your time to make a list of your functional limitations before visiting your physician rather than trusting your memory.

You can apply for benefits by calling or visiting your local Social Security office. They will take information over the telephone and send you an application, or they may give you an appointment to come in for an interview. All of the items on the application forms are important and should be completed carefully. You should be prepared to furnish accurate names, addressees, and telephone numbers (including facsimile numbers) of your physicians, hospitals, and therapists. The specific dates of treatment and the exact type of treatment or tests you have had are also important. A list of the medications that you take, along with an explanation of why you are taking them, can be beneficial. You will also be asked to provide the dates and descriptions of all jobs you have held for the past 15 years.

The disability adjudication process is actually much more complex than this brief summary might indicate. You can obtain more details by accessing the SSA Web site at http://www.ssa.gov. (Find the header "Benefits Information" and click on disability.) Information is also available through the SSA hotline at 800-772-1213. Service representatives are on duty from 7 A.M. to 7 P.M., and recorded information is available 24 hours per day. You can obtain the booklet *Disability Benefits* (Publication 05-10029) by calling or visiting any Social Security office.

CHAPTER 14

Restless Legs Syndrome and Relationships

O NE OF THE MOST DIFFICULT ASPECTS of living with RLS is its affect on relationships. The discomfort, fatigue, and restrictions caused by RLS can spill over into your relationships, making it impossible to maintain intimate or close associations. Do you stay home by yourself instead of going to the movies or a restaurant? Do you find yourself sleeping on

> One of the most difficult aspects of living with RLS is its affect on relationships.

the couch or in a separate bed some or all of the time? Have you turned down a dinner invitation, a party, or a date? Maybe you have stopped doing things you used to do with others. If so, you probably already know the affect of RLS on your relationships.

People use many strategies to help keep their relationships healthy when faced with a chronic disorder such as RLS. Educating yourself and the other people in your life are important. Managing RLS to ensure improved quality of life is also important. If you can lessen the time RLS symptoms plague you, there will be fewer disruptions in your relationships.

Ann Battenfield, who has lived with RLS for a long time and knows the toll RLS can take on a relationship, has written the rest of this chapter.

How RLS Disrupts Relationships

Restrictions

"I feel trapped in my home and in my own body," says one young woman with severe RLS. Having RLS often means being restricted in many areas of your life, including social life with family and friends, which can lead to stress or feelings of anger, frustration, or grief.

People with RLS often avoid activities that require sitting, especially during the evening hours. Many shared activities involve sitting, such as watching a movie, car rides, plane trips, or going out to dinner. These restrictions create a difficult situation for both the person with RLS and for those close to them. Lee, a 45-year-old man with severe PLMD, echoes the sentiments of many when he says, "Your social life becomes optional when you are fatigued and can barely complete simple tasks, such as going to work or feeding the children." If you have a long-standing card game with a group of friends every Friday evening, you might stop going. If this was the primary time you spent with these friends, your friendships will probably be affected.

The restrictions of RLS can take a toll on your sex life, too. People have less desire to have sex when they are exhausted. The medications for RLS can affect desire, functioning, and mood. People with severe RLS often find themselves sleeping in different beds from their partners, which is where many couples initiate sex. These restrictions are often frustrating. When a loved one has a problem, the first efforts may be to find a solution, but RLS cannot be "solved," and it may take time for the person with RLS to gain control of the disorder.

Liz and Drew were taken by surprise when her RLS suddenly became much worse. The medications were not working, and Liz was sleeping less than 3 hours a night. Anxious, stressed, and feeling like she was never going to get better, she started crying one morning. Drew immediately became angry and walked into the next room saying, "I can't take this." After they had calmed down and were able to talk about it, Drew admitted that he was not angry with Liz, nor did her crying anger him. He was frustrated because there was nothing he could do. He felt impotent to help her. As one person with RLS pointed out, "There is no bandage for RLS, which gives our spouse or partner little opportunity to help."

It can be difficult to create and maintain relationships when faced with the restrictions of RLS. You might avoid starting a new relationship if you do not think someone will tolerate the restrictions you might need to place on it. Restrictions on sex and other activities can weaken a relationship, possibly resulting in a break-up or divorce. Other activities, such as taking a vacation, can be extremely difficult financially and physically when you cannot stay in a family member's house or share a hotel room without disrupting those around you.

Some people with RLS may consider not having children, even if they want them. Women have additional difficulties. During pregnancy they cannot take most of the RLS drugs, and RLS symptoms are often much worse during pregnancy. After braving one pregnancy, some women may decide that they cannot go through another, no matter how many children they would like to have. For men or women who are managing severe RLS, the thought of taking care of young children may seem too difficult when coupled with RLS symptoms. For people with a family history of RLS, there may be concerns of passing RLS on to their children.

Loss

Anger, resentment, misunderstandings, and guilt often accompany the experience of loss. Ilene found out about this when, in her 50s, she began dating a man who cooked romantic dinners, seemed to adore being with her, and pampered her in many other ways. She felt deeply loved and cared for when they were together. After a few months, they decided to share an apartment. On nights when her RLS was active, she would sleep on the couch. The next morning her boyfriend would accuse her of not wanting to be with him and not loving him.

Loss of sleep is extremely common in RLS. Any household member can lose sleep because of the constant awakenings, movement, and nocturnal wandering of the person with RLS. The bed partner may lose sleep and may choose to sleep in another bed. This may resolve some of the problems, but it also removes a primary source of physical contact and intimacy. Loss of intimacy in close relationships between couples, family, or close friends is devastating to everyone involved. Intimacy, as talked about here in relation to RLS, includes both physical and emotional closeness. For example, you may lose physical closeness, such as snuggling or sitting together on the couch while watching TV, because it could trigger an RLS attack.

Emotional closeness can suffer if you do not talk about your RLS experience. Relationships also suffer if you talk about your experience and do not feel that the other person believes or understands you. It is common to feel that no one understands your problems. There is no shared language to explain RLS, and a feeling of deep and persistent loneliness can result. Misunderstandings, denial, and lack of open communication erode intimacy. They can also build mistrust, anger, and frustration. The changes caused by a chronic disorder such as RLS can be particularly stressful. Both parties may question how much they will lose, including their plans, dreams, and hopes. Sleep deprivation and medications sometimes have a dramatic effect on how people feel, therefore affecting how they act. If this happens, you may wonder what is wrong with you, and your partner may feel like the person he fell in love with has been lost.

RLS sometimes causes the loss of a partner's understanding and compassion. They may become annoyed and lose patience with the foot-tapping, arm-waving, or other movements that are necessary to eliminate uncomfortable sensations. It is extremely difficult to explain how this disorder feels or why moving the affected body part is unavoidable. RLS has not received much attention, and few people know anything about it. It is similar to other "invisible" disorders. You may appear healthy to your friends, coworkers, and family because there are no physical signs to reveal how fatigued or ill you feel.

There may also be financial considerations. People with severe RLS might have to change jobs, work less, or stop working completely. They may be unable to contribute financially, as they did in the past. The loss of income and inability to meet joint financial goals can cause additional strains.

Fear

Fear often accompanies restrictions and loss, and this can be a major barrier to acceptance and understanding. Emotions such as anger and frustration often accompany fear, leading to stress and depression. Fear of the future is common. Stephen, in his 20s and with refractory RLS, says that he wishes he were already old. He worries that his RLS will worsen and *always* affect his life. His fiancée finds these thoughts distressing and wonders what type of future they can have together.

People with RLS sometimes fear being alone in the future. Will their current partner stay with them? Will anyone want them? They may wonder if they will ever get better and how they can continue living without relief. There may be concerns about medication. What are the side effects? What if their current medication is no longer effective?

Sharing the details of how RLS affects you can be terrifying. You have to decide whom to tell, how much to tell, when to tell, and how to ask for support. Fear is associated with sharing for a good reason. You can never be sure of the response, and you might not get the response you want. Some people will not be able to support you, regardless of your need. Holly, who was misdiagnosed with depression and put on drugs that made her RLS worse, still struggles with RLS and chronic fatigue syndrome. "My family knows I don't sleep, but they don't really *know*."

You may be afraid that people will see you differently if you tell them about your RLS. One man thought his wife would think he was broken or inferior if he told her how much RLS affects him. Friends and family often do not like hearing about physical problems, because it conjures up images and thoughts of mortality and vulnerability. You may fear the loss of your independence. If your RLS symptoms or medication restricts your ability to drive, how will you get around? Will you be able to work? How will your family, spouse, or partner feel about helping you? You might fear that you will not meet your goals.

The people in your life might fear the inevitable losses that will occur over time. They may fear that you are overreacting or taking advantage of the situation. This often leads to anger and resentment. Your partner may also fear that he or she is not strong enough to help or will not be able to meet your needs.

Taking RLS Seriously

The resulting attitudes, feelings, and responses to restrictions, loss, and fear can create difficulties in any relationship. There are additional problems that can prevent people from taking your problems with RLS seriously. Perhaps you have said something like "I know I shouldn't complain. It isn't like RLS is terminal." RLS may not be terminal, but it is chronic and can cause disruptions in your life and your relationships. Comparing yourself to others can cause you to minimize your problems, preventing you from finding solutions.

Other people might minimize your problems inadvertently because they think it will help you feel better. Some people lack understanding. Good sleepers cannot imagine how difficult it can be to fall asleep. They may not take you seriously, especially if your physician has dismissed your RLS problems.

WHAT YOU CAN DO

How can you take a vacation with your family? What can you do to prevent emotional disconnection from your partner or family? What should you say when someone asks you about RLS? How can you keep intimacy in your life and prevent your relationship from ending because of the disruptions caused by RLS? As discussed in Chapter 12, coping strategies can provide solutions, but ongoing disruptions from RLS can eventually cause problems in relationships. Good communication skills can prevent this from happening.

Communication Basics

Effective communication is essential for healthy relationships. The affects of RLS can hamper effective communication, even in the happiest and healthiest relationships. Direct, honest communication, done in a caring way, can help you maintain your relationships when your RLS is out of control and may help you form stronger relationships when your RLS is under control.

There are many on relationships and communication (see Appendix). Read these books, attend workshops, or see a professional counselor to help develop you communication skills. Remember, both parties must be willing to participate for success in relationships. In his book *Will Our Love Last?*, Sam Hamburg explains that all successful relationships have an underlying element of *respect*. Understanding and

> Effective communication is essential for healthy relationships.

compassion will be lacking if there is no respect. This can create communication problems, especially in relationships that include a person who has a chronic condition such as RLS. Mutual respect is also the basis for friendships. If you find yourself saying or hearing, "Why did he do *that*? He knows how much RLS bothers me!" or, "I just don't understand why she just can't sit still," you are having problems with respect.

Respect occurs naturally when people share a common attitude regarding issues important to them. People with RLS usually provide immediate understanding and compassion to one another; however, what can you do when those around you do not have RLS? Identify a problem the other person has or something that creates difficulty for them. You might choose a medical problem. You can use this as an analogy to help them understand how your RLS affects you. For example, you can say something like "Do you remember when you told me how your life is affected when you have anxiety attacks? You can't sleep, you're tired, you feel like no one understands, and you think it will never feel better? RLS affects me the same way."

Offer unconditional respect, even if you do not understand what someone with RLS is going through. The fact that you care about this person is all you need to do this. When someone important to you says that their quality of life is affected by RLS, do your best to believe it. It should make no difference whether or not you can understand what they are actually experiencing.

The people in your life will not understand of what you are experiencing unless you tell them. *Sharing* helps creates intimacy. Lynne, who has had RLS for a long time, said, "I never realized how much of the RLS truth I hid from those who really care about me. Maybe knowing the facts gives people close to me the opportunity to make life easier."

Fear prevents us from sharing, including the fear that you have already burdened others enough. "I thought he knew what I meant when I said *pain*," Lynne said sheepishly. "When I finally got brave enough to say, 'I need to talk,' I was shocked at how little he knew about what I was going through. He did not know that I was afraid to drive because I was not alert enough, or that I didn't watch TV with him because it was so uncomfortable. He deserved better from me. I think I am moving in the right direction now, ever so slowly, but moving forward."

Guidelines for Sharing

You can share a little, or a lot. You can share all at once, or once in awhile. Decide whom and how much to tell. Tell only the people who need to know. The closer and more intimate the relationship, the more you should tell. Keeping secrets about RLS will create difficulties when the other person eventually finds out.

Set boundaries, as needed. If you are not used to sharing with a particular person or have had difficulties with them in the past, discuss the process ahead of time. Explain that this is difficult for you and ask them to be respectful. Ask them to listen without judgment. You may also want to ask them to keep the conversation confidential. Allow enough time for this important conversation about your RLS. Stress that you want to avoid interruptions. Set a specific time to prevent other activities from interfering.

Identify the purpose of sharing and expected outcomes. Why do you want to share? What do you hope to get out of it? You can think of these as your *goals*; however, goals must be things you can control. You cannot control what another person does, thinks, or says. You may want to "make her understand," however her understanding is not something you can control. You can only control the way you explain RLS. What do you want the person to know about your RLS? How can they help you or the situation? How can you explain RLS in a way that they will understand? What problems need to be resolved? Think of analogies, examples, or other ways that may help the other person understand your difficulties with RLS.

Consider sharing in a support group environment or with a counselor if you need assistance. This can lessen the strain on your existing relationships. Your partner or best friend may be compassionate and understanding; however, he or she may not want or be able to spend the amount of time you need to discuss your symptoms, medications, and concerns.

Be clear about your purpose and expectations. Allow time for both of you to explain what is important. You can start by sharing your perspective, or by asking how the other person feels. Ask for whatever you want—you may not get it, but your chances will be better if you are explicit. You can ask for help to resolve a specific problem or with the whole situation. Be open to all suggestions, even if an idea sounds ridiculous or stupid when you first hear it. Not all ideas may work as initially offered, but parts of them might. Creativity is stifled when you rush to judgment during the process.

In any relationship, both parties need to agree on how to resolve issues. You may request something that will help you, but what if that request causes resentment? Agree to a solution that you both find acceptable and that neither of you will resent. Be specific about dates, times, or other details, because it will prevent misunderstandings later.

Listening requires your undivided attention. Concentrate on the other person's words *and* their tone of voice and posture. Do not concentrate on the solution, your own side of the story, or questions. It is easier not to judge or interrupt when you listen from a place of respect. Use your body language to show that you are listening; for example, make eye contact, face the other person, and nod in understanding. When someone speaks, let them know you are listening. You can "restate" or repeat exactly what you heard them say. (It is best to use this technique infrequently.) An example would be:

He: "I want us to work harder to find a solution!"
You: "You want us to work harder to find a solution."

You can state in your own words what you though you heard the other person say. Use this technique more frequently than the restating technique. For example:

She: "What have we done about this in the past? We talk about it and do nothing. We just haven't worked hard enough. I need more than that."

You: "I heard you say that you don't feel we've worked hard enough in the past on finding a solution, and that it is important for to you for us to work harder in the future."

You can also summarize occasionally. It can be helpful to ask the person if you heard them correctly, for example:

He: "This is so difficult. We don't do any of the things we used to do. Do you remember when we used to go out with Brenda and Chris? We don't ever see them anymore! They still do things together, and they sure seem happier than we are."

You: "Let me make sure I understand what you said. You are worried about our relationship because we don't do the things we used to do. Is that right?"

Welcome emotional expression, even though some emotions can be unpleasant or frightening. Acknowledging a person's feelings allows them to let go of those feelings and concentrate on solutions. It can be hard to acknowledge emotions, and it is even harder when respect is lacking. We may find ourselves judging, either the person or the emotion. We might say, "You shouldn't feel that way," or "What a horrible thing to think!" Instead, try to respect the other person's perspective, even if it is not the same as your own. You can nod or touch the other person's arm if you do not know what to say, or you can acknowledge the emotion by saying: "I can hear in your voice how upsetting this is for you." If you are not sure how a person feels, ask.

Be specific. Explain exactly how you feel and offer examples. For instance, say you are talking to your best friend. She is hurt and angry because you canceled your dinner plans the last three times. When explaining why you canceled, you say, "It's because I have a lot of pain." But, will she understand what you are saying? What does "a lot of pain" mean?

You might say instead, "Each day I have to drag myself out of bed; I feel constant fatigue that lasts all day. I can never think clearly. I'm always in a fog and rarely feel bright and cheery. Rather I'm down in the dumps. But it's the evenings that are worst. When someone suggests going out to a movie or having dinner together, I almost never accept, because I know that I will suffer through the whole thing, constantly moving my feet and aching to get up and walk out of the theater or restaurant. I can't really enjoy any such social event." This kind of in-depth communication can promote richer and fuller understanding in a relationship.

A person cannot help you if she does not know what you need. If someone said to you, "This is horrible. I am so unhappy. I do not like it at all," would you know what they needed? Maybe the person is venting. Maybe they need something but are not telling you in specific terms. If you are missing intimacy, say you are missing intimacy. If you have a need, state it; for example, you could say: "I cannot get up in the morning in time to walk the dog and get ready for work because I was up most of the night with RLS. Will you help me?" Specific statements indicate both the problem and the request for help.

Create a safe environment. Emotional and physical safety is important. For most people, "safe" means they feel free from harm, welcomed, respected, and free to express their needs. People who encounter sarcasm, demeaning statements, criticism, or privacy violations are less likely to feel safe. Sharing honestly and openly requires feeling safe.

Be open to new ideas or solutions. There is a saying, "If you always do what you've always done, you'll always get what you've always got." Solving problems may require creativity. Do things differently. Reassign roles and responsibilities. Be flexible. Try not to dismiss new ideas. Say, "That's an interesting idea," instead of, "No." Try saying, "I thought about it before. Maybe I will think about it again," instead of, "Yes, but it won't work because . . ." Not all new ideas will work, but sometimes parts of them will. Combining strategies can produce a better solution.

Liz and Drew live in a one-bedroom loft condominium and share a king-sized bed. When her medication lost its effectiveness, she was either moving in bed or getting up and down many times throughout the night. Liz found it difficult to navigate the dark stairway, but Drew

> Be open to new ideas or solutions.

could not sleep with light in the room. Drew experienced frequent awakenings from the movement of the mattress. Liz ended up on the couch in order to make it easier for both of them. They soon felt the loss of intimacy to which they were accustomed. They did not have a second bed, the couch was uncomfortable, and they wanted to be together at night. But how? They thought of many ideas before settling on a final solution.

They decided on twin beds put together to form one large bed. Because the frames and mattresses were separate, neither felt the other's movements and they could sleep together. They installed a nightlight at the bottom of the stairs that was bright enough for Liz to see and far enough away from the bedroom so it did not bother Drew. He began wearing earplugs so her footsteps during the night did not awaken him.

Working Together to Stay Together

Effective communication is an important way to keep relationships healthy. Other strategies can provide solutions to the disruptions of RLS and help relationships at the same time. Communication can take place in ways other than talking face-to-face. A few months after she decided to share the "honest truth" about her RLS with her husband, Lynn came up with the idea of interviewing him. She asked him to spend some time with her sharing what he observed and his experience with her RLS. He saw her sleeping, so who better to ask? He was able to provide details that she never would have known. She found out how much she moved at night, how these movements affected him, and how worried he had been about her.

Similarly, Nick asked his wife to write a letter to him about how his RLS affected her life. He had tried to hide it from her for several years, refusing to talk about it in detail. He was afraid she would see him as less of a man and a husband than when she had married him. Over time, his RLS worsened and their relationship became strained. When he finally realized that he needed her support and help, he knew he needed to be more open with her. He was worried about how his RLS was affecting her. However, he was too afraid to hear her response directly and asked for a letter instead. The sharing of the letter was emotional and cathartic for both of them. He found that he had never completely hidden it from her. In fact, his attempts at hiding it had created the strain in their relationship, not the RLS itself.

Lynne and Nick each found a way to help their spouses become an ally. They used adversity to become closer and create more intimacy. You can do this with the people in any of your close relationships; for example, you can ask for a letter from your best friend or sister. You could also send a letter to your parents or your adult children. Another way to communicate to those close to you is in a support group. Hearing other people's stories, problems, and solutions often provides a new way of looking at your own. In addition, people who do *not* have RLS can learn about it by attending these meetings.

When needed, change your priorities. As soon as a strategy stops working, identify new solutions. Do not let disruptions continue. Remain vigilant about identifying the restrictions, losses, and fears that cause disruptions. Some couples decide to sleep in separate beds, or even separate rooms, but they make time each morning for a few minutes of physical contact in the form of a hug and a kiss.

If you are looking for a long-term relationship, carefully consider at which point to discuss your RLS. If you cannot participate in cuddling, snuggling, or sleeping in the same bed, decide when you will tell your prospective partner. Some people believe in discussing it immediately; others prefer to wait until they see the potential for a lasting relationship. The longer you wait to tell someone, the greater the chance that your partner will be resentful. Whenever you decide to discuss your RLS, it is helpful to express your willingness to find other ways to create a sense of closeness.

COPING SKILLS

In her book *Sleep Thief, Restless Legs Syndrome*, Virginia Wilson writes, "A happy marriage is not proof of how compatible the partners are, but proof of how the partners cope with incompatibility." This applies to all successful relationships, not just marriage or intimate relationships.

You may need to set limits or boundaries on activities. These limits may include consistency in the time you go to bed, taking your medications on time, or avoiding going places that require a late-night car, bus, or train ride home. Knowing what activates your RLS will allow you to have more freedom overall and participate in activities you previously avoided; for example, you might decide o change your Friday night card game to Sunday afternoon.

Schedule a time for intimacy. Liz and Drew found that sex and snuggling never happened spontaneously. "Drew loves to snuggle, either at night before sleep or in the morning when we wake up. He started complaining that we never did it anymore. Well, he goes to bed at 10:00 P.M., and I often don't go to bed until 2:00 A.M. We were never in bed at the same time!"

Liz first thought of offering to snuggle with Drew at his bedtime. "Once in awhile, I would ask him at bedtime if he wanted company. If he said yes, I would get into bed with him, snuggle until he fell asleep, and then get up." Soon, they started discussing which night would work best that week. When Drew's work schedule allowed, he started offering to "sleep in" until Liz was awake, at which time they could snuggle. They tend to schedule only a day or two in advance. They know they might have to reschedule when Liz is struggling with RLS symptoms. They work together to choose a day and time that works best. Since scheduling snuggling was so successful, they began to schedule sex, too. "Before we started scheduling sex, sometimes two months would go by before it would happen spontaneously. We are much closer now," Liz said.

You may find yourself isolated and spending more time alone when RLS is severe. You may feel angry, depressed, or frustrated when you are fatigued, having trouble working, or not able to communicate clearly. At these times, do the best you can to stay involved, even if on a limited basis. People who cut themselves off from others are more prone to depression. It is also harder to manage your RLS when you feel isolated and alone.

"I have severe RLS. The fatigue prevents me from regularly seeing my friends." Emma has not worked for almost 2 years and is fighting for disability. Instead of losing her friends, as you might think, she has maintained close relationships with them. "Friendships cannot survive with one-way traffic. Both parties have to stay involved. I talk on the phone with them, which is good, because I hear their voices and we can laugh. However, my best asset in this isolated situation is e-mail. I am lucky that so many of my friends and ex-colleagues send me long e-mails that bring me up to date about their life and work. These e-mails give me so much pleasure that I honestly think this kind of communication is almost as good as face-to-face contact. Answering their posts makes me happy and gives me a feeling of closeness. E-mail is my window to the world of my friends and relatives."

Be as flexible as you can. When difficulties arise, flexibility is usually one of the faster routes to a solution; for example, imagine your kids are mad at you because you do not visit them. Of course, the real reason is that you are not comfortable staying in their house because of your RLS.

> Be flexible and keep your sense of humor.

You could use effective communication to improve your relationship with your kids, but you could also use flexibility to find a way to visit them. This provides a short-term solution for the problem. Perhaps you could rent an RV and park it in front of their house or find a hotel/motel to ensure an enjoyable visit.

Maintaining a sense of humor is another way to cope with the disruptions of RLS and keep balance in your relationships. Humor can be hard to come by when you are in the midst of a sleepless night. When possible, take a deep breath and find something humorous about the situation. Studies have shown that laughter contributes to emotional and physical health.

CHAPTER 15

Finding a Physician

F INDING THE RIGHT PHYSICIAN can be one of the most difficult tasks facing a person with RLS. What makes this so difficult is that most physicians know little, if anything about RLS. Many health care professionals think that RLS is not even a real disease! The reason that most physicians have limited knowledge about RLS is that they have received almost no education on the subject. Most medical school curriculums contain only a short reference to RLS during an allotted 1-hour lecture on sleep. Some medical schools have recently added a 1-hour lecture on RLS.

Having no FDA-approved drug for RLS until recently has also hampered the ability to treat this disorder. Many physicians feel uncomfortable prescribing drugs for *off-label* (non–FDA approved) use. Physicians who might prescribe these drugs are not able to find prescription guidelines, and this lack of information has preventing many willing physicians from treating RLS.

Pharmaceutical companies cannot sponsor seminars about the use of a drug for treating RLS until the FDA approves it for that specific disease. With the May 2005 FDA approval of ropinirole as the first RLS drug— and hopefully several more are on the way—many more RLS educational opportunities are now available. However, it will likely take a few more years before the majority of physicians gain the knowledge and comfort level necessary to manage RLS successfully.

PRIMARY CARE PHYSICIANS

Most people with RLS do not need to see a specialist. Any competent and caring primary care physician should be able to treat your RLS symptoms. Although most of them are not knowledgeable about RLS, they are learning, and many should be ready to treat RLS properly in the near future. Your personal physician is the best choice to treat your RLS if he or she is up to date on the available information. However, even if this is not the case, it does not necessarily mean that you should look elsewhere for treatment. Make an appointment with your physician and discuss whether he or she is willing to treat your RLS.

Some physicians are eager to learn new areas of medicine; others are not. As discussed in previous chapters, working with your physician as a team will help in the management of RLS. Supply your physician with the appropriate RLS medical literature, as listed in the Appendix. For most people with mild to moderate RLS, teaming up with your primary care physician can easily result in successful treatment. If your primary care physician is unwilling to manage your RLS, search for another primary physician who is willing to treat you.

Many smaller communities do not have medical specialists; often primary care physicians cover these gaps. Using current reference material, including the Mayo Clinic Proceedings RLS Algorithm (see Appendix), primary physicians who are motivated should easily be able to treat most people with mild to moderate RLS.

Primary care physicians often do not manage patients with RLS appropriately. Understanding why may help enable you to get proper care for your RLS. Many of the problems encountered with primary care physicians stem from the busy nature of their practices and their lack of knowledge about RLS. Medical practices are demanding and keeping current with all areas of medicine can be a daunting task. It is much easier for physicians to update their knowledge about a disease that they already know fairly well. Learning about a new disorder such as RLS is a much more difficult task. Fortunately, physicians will become more knowledgeable as the opportunities to learn about RLS increase.

You can help educate your physician about RLS. Bring informational pamphlets, articles, or this book with you to an office visit. By highlighting the sections that pertain to your particular problem, you can focus your physician's attention on possible treatments. This can be an efficient and effective way to use your physician's limited time. Most physicians will appreciate your efforts. To get the best results, approach your physician tactfully, rather than demanding that he or she follow the advice given in the literature. After you build up some trust in this process, it will be easier for your physician to institute the therapies suggested by your sources.

RLS SPECIALISTS

People with more severe or refractory RLS may need a higher level of expertise. Some primary care physicians have taken a real interest in RLS and have experience treating this disorder, but if an appropriate primary care doctor is not available in your area, obtain a referral to a specialist. Sleep specialists and neurologists have the most expertise in treating RLS. However, even when choosing a physician from these two specialties, you should make sure that the specialist treats many people with RLS and has knowledge to treat more difficult cases. Neurologists who specialize in movement disorders, such as Parkinson's disease, often are better qualified to treat severe RLS.

Asking your regular physician for a referral to an RLS specialist should be the easiest way to find appropriate treatment. Unfortunately, most primary care physicians have not yet established a referral network for people with RLS, and it is likely that your physician will refer you to the local neurologist or sleep specialist. You must still ascertain whether the specialist is capable of treating difficult cases of RLS. This may not be an easy task, because, typically, the only way to verify the specialist's competence in RLS may be to see how well he or she treats your case.

How can you determine a specialist's ability to treat RLS before making an appointment? You can ask your primary physician how many cases the specialist has treated and whether the outcomes were successful. This strategy works only with primary physicians who have some experience with referring difficult cases. Most often the burden of finding an RLS specialist falls upon the patient. One method is to call the specialist's office yourself and speak to the office staff. They can usually tell you how many difficult RLS cases the physician sees and what drugs he or she uses for treatment. This may give you some insight into whether the physician really has the expertise to treat severe RLS.

The RLS Foundation maintains on their Web site (see Appendix) a list of physicians who are willing to treat RLS. These physicians are interested in treating people with RLS, although their expertise is not certain. They may range from a national expert to someone who has seen only one or two RLS cases. This list is an appropriate starting place, especially for people who live in rural or other medically underserviced areas and need to find a physician.

> The best way to find a specialist with the expertise to treat RLS is to ask other people with RLS.

The best way to find a specialist with the expertise to treat RLS is to ask other people with RLS. Members of your local support group should be able to direct you to an experienced physician. Internet-based support groups, forums, and bulletin boards can also be helpful. People with RLS who live in rural areas should be prepared to travel significant distances to see a specialist.

Most people should be able to find a competent physician to treat their RLS by using these suggestions. However, a small percentage of people with severe and refractory RLS may be beyond the ability of the available physicians. These people should try to arrange a consultation with one of the national RLS specialists. You can find these higher-level specialists in several ways. Your local physician may be able to help you find one, and the Web-based RLS community is well aware of these physicians and can direct you to several of them. Another source is the RLS Foundation, which sponsors RLS meetings and can give you the names of the physicians who speak at these meetings. You can also find physicians who publish medical articles on RLS by doing a literature search using the free PubMed service (see Appendix).

There is no guarantee that any national specialist will be able to treat your RLS more successfully than your local RLS specialist, but it is worth a try. If all of the currently available treatments are of no benefit, the specialist might know of a clinical trial that employs a new type of therapy. You can also look for clinical trials yourself on the RLS Foundation's Web site. Keep in mind, however, that there is usually a 50 percent chance that you will be assigned to the placebo (sugar pill) study group. In addition, most drug studies require you to stop all your regular RLS medications and spend a week or longer without taking any medication.

How to Work with Your Physician

It can be intimidating when people sense that their physicians are busy. Treatment of RLS must compete with the management of their more commonly accepted medical problems, such as high blood pressure, diabetes, or high cholesterol. Below are typical quotes from people who have experienced this problem:

"I am going to see my doctor in 2 days and I'm worried. I have only a few minutes to state my case and make him realize how miserable I am."

"My physician is so busy; I don't want to bother him."

People often wait until after their physician has finished addressing their other problems before bringing up RLS. Most busy primary care physicians schedule only 10–15 minutes for follow-up visits, which includes time to write prescriptions and chart notes. By the time the RLS concerns are brought up, many physicians already have their hand on the doorknob and are ready to move on to their next patient. This is clearly not the right time to initiate a prolonged discussion on RLS!

Try scheduling a separate visit for the sole purpose of discussing RLS. When making this appointment, indicate that you need an extended time slot (usually 20–30 minutes or longer) for the visit. These planned, longer visits should avoid stressing your physician for time, thus allowing him or her to listen to your RLS complaints and address them.

There are only two acceptable outcomes from an extended RLS appointment: your physician will (1) agree to treat your RLS or (2) refer you to another physician with more expertise. Any other result is unacceptable. If your physician says, "There is no such disease as RLS and your problems are all in your head," or "You are just anxious and need to relax," you may have an insurmountable problem with that physician. If after reading the literature on RLS and hearing your RLS history your physician still does not acknowledge your disorder, you should consider looking for another physician.

Your physician may still misdiagnose your disorder, despite your best efforts. You must be prepared to act if he or she she tries to prescribe a medication such as quinine for leg cramps, an anti-inflammatory drug for arthritis, or an antidepressant for depression. Taking these drugs will not help your RLS and may even worsen the problem. You should refuse to take them and point out that you really do have RLS. It may be helpful to give your physician a copy of the four key RLS diagnostic criteria (see Chapter 2) and discuss how you fulfill these criteria. If this proactive approach upsets your physician and prevents you from getting treatment for your RLS, you should consider finding another physician.

How to Get the Right Medication

People with RLS must become well educated about drug use in RLS and then educate their physicians. This means doing your homework in advance. As discussed above, do not accept a drug that does not work for RLS or that tends to worsen it. Another problem may arise with physicians who have looked up the treatment of RLS in their textbooks (which usually contain information that is a few years out of date, even when published) and prescribe a medication such as levodopa for daily RLS, which will eventually worsen the disorder. Come prepared with credible literature that supports the use of effective RLS drugs and discusses how to use them. Highlight the sections that pertain directly to your situation.

Another problem often arises with the use of narcotics, which can be the only effective RLS drugs for some people. Many physicians feel uncomfortable about prescribing them, particularly long term. Some may prescribe the less potent schedule 3 drugs (codeine, hydrocodone, and propoxyphene) but not the more potent schedule 2 drugs (levorphanol, methadone, and oxycodone). People with RLS have said: "Trying to get my physician to prescribe hydrocodone, and in a sufficient dose, is like pulling teeth" or "My physician called me a junkie."

You can discuss the general safety of these medications in RLS—when monitored carefully—and support this with medical literature. However, if your physician still does not feel at ease with prescribing these medications, there is likely nothing you can do to change his or her mind. You will need a referral to a specialist or find another primary care physician who will prescribe them.

INSURANCE COVERAGE FOR RLS

Obtaining health insurance is often a significant concern for those people with RLS who do not have any, have just lost their insurance coverage, or wish to change it. It is usually easy to get health insurance when you are part of a large group such as a business with many employees. Health insurance companies rarely reject members of large groups, although they may charge somewhat higher fees to those with significant health problems.

However, it is definitely not easy for people who are not members of these large groups to acquire health insurance. This includes people who work for themselves, in small businesses, or part-time. Having RLS does not guarantee that insurance companies will reject you, but it does increase that risk.

Every health insurance company has different criteria for accepting or rejecting members, which may also vary by state. Rejection may only occur when other underlying problems are present in addition to RLS. These other problems need not be active ones. They might include conditions such as asthma that was only present as a child, controlled high blood pressure, controlled high cholesterol, or a remote history of migraine headaches. Despite the fact that these medical conditions are far in the past or currently controlled, they still count these as strikes against you. Depending on the insurance company, two, three, or four strikes against you are sufficient to reject your bid for insurance or to increase your fees dramatically. Having your physician or other health professional write a letter explaining that the previous or current medical conditions present no increased risk is of no benefit. Insurance companies have incredibly rigid rules and make their decisions based only on actuarial tables, not on any supportive letters. Life insurance and long-term disability insurance companies often use these same criteria to reject or accept applicants (see Appendix).

What do you do when your insurance does not cover your RLS drug? This can be a problem because so far only one medication, ropinirole, is FDA approved for RLS. Most insurance companies will approve and pay for a drug that is not FDA approved for RLS once there have been two peer-reviewed research studies published in accepted medical journals supporting the use of the drug in RLS.

Insurance companies might place other roadblocks in the way of getting RLS drugs. They can require prior authorization before they will agree to cover drugs that are not on their list of covered drugs or ones that are covered but have higher co-payments. To get prior authorization, your physician must fill out a form (sometimes even two or three) explaining why you need the drug and why you are unable to benefit from the other drugs that are on the approved list. Many busy physicians resent the extra time and effort necessary to fill out this paperwork, and they may need some prodding to expedite the drug approval. You must be proactive while waiting for drug approval by your insurance company. Be persistent but polite with your physician's office staff. This is often a situation where the squeaky wheel gets the grease.

Working with Your HMO

It may be more difficult for people covered under an HMO (health maintenance organization) to follow the above-described suggestions regarding prescriptions. People covered under HMOs cannot self-refer, but rather must get a referral from their primary care physician, which often needs further approval by an authorization committee. They must go through the HMO system to see an RLS specialist—or pay cash to see the specialist as a non-covered service. If you are an HMO patient and your primary care physician refuses to refer you to an RLS specialist, you still have some options.

One option is to change to another primary care physician within your HMO. Make sure the new physician will either treat your RLS or refer you to a specialist. Changing to another physician may take some time, further delaying your treatment. Another option is to petition your HMO for a consultation with an RLS specialist. This may take several telephone calls and letters, but if you are persistent you should be successful.

What do you do if there is no RLS specialist on your HMO's panel who is capable enough to treat your RLS? This may seem like a dead end to many people with RLS, but there still is hope. HMOs must provide a specialist that can manage your medical problem. If they do not have one in their specialist network, they must pay for a physician outside the network. This process often takes quite a while, and requires many telephone calls, letters, and lots of time filling forms. It is not surprising that many people with HMOs simply elect to find a competent RLS specialist and pay out-of-pocket.

CHAPTER 16

The Future of Restless Legs Syndrome Treatment

WHAT CAN WE FORESEE for the future of RLS? In many ways we are just emerging from the dark ages in the understanding of RLS, and many readers will agree that they have suffered through these dark ages. But now there is a bit of light and hope, and perhaps more will come in the near future. What gives us hope? The scientific literature on RLS doubles roughly every 5 years, but the data on clinical trial reports are even more dramatic. The articles on RLS published in 2004 and 2005 included more information than had been reported in all of the previous literature. Those of us who were aware of or studying RLS in the 1980s can scarcely believe how much progress has been made.

ADVANCES IN TREATMENT

As discussed throughout this book, the first drug to be approved for use in RLS in the U.S. was ropinirole (Requip®), which was approved in May 2005, and soon thereafter in Europe. Pramipexole (Mirapex™) is now also approved in Europe, with approval pending in the United States as of July 2006. A levodopa compound, levodopa and benser-azide (Restex®), had already been approved a few years earlier in Europe within selected countries. This was a tremendous advance, because having a drug approved qualifies it for inclusion in the *PDR*, making it easier for physicians to prescribe it. Approval puts RLS in the medical mainstream. Now that the ice has been broken and one drug is approved, others will surely follow. Several companies are seeking to get

213

other drugs approved for RLS, and we can expect that these drugs will also be dopamine agonists, which are recognized as the drugs of choice for daily RLS.

Other types of drugs are expected to follow. Anticonvulsants such as gabapentin (Neurontin®), but probably not gabapentin itself, may be early candidates. Narcotics may also be approved for RLS; at least, most RLS experts hope so, because these are excellent drugs for many people with RLS. They can be given at many different dosages and with many different durations of action. They seem to offer some special advantage for truly refractory patients. If RLS proves to be a useful market for the drug companies, other ideas may be developed and completely different drugs—beyond those discussed in this book—may be tried for RLS.

The development of dopamine-enhancing medications similar to those now available, but with a longer half-life, is expected. Such drugs may help the problem of augmentation, which is an occasionally nasty stumbling block in the treatment of daily RLS. As already mentioned, augmentation may be caused by the rapid rise and fall of medication levels in the blood and brain that occurs with drugs having a shorter duration of action. Cabergoline is a model for these long-acting drugs.

Another development may be the greater application of drugs that do not need to be taken by mouth. Some of these drugs have already been tested, if only on a few people. One drug that is likely to be available soon is rotigotine. This drug is undergoing large-scale trials and has been developed for delivery using a skin patch. One report says it works quite well. Rotigotine offers the possibility of keeping an even level of drug in the body, which may also make a difference with augmentation. Another drug soon to follow is lisuride; both are dopamine agonists. Apomorphine (Apokyn®) has recently been approved in the U.S. for Parkinson's disease. It is both a dopamine agonist and a narcotic that is given subcutaneously, meaning with a shot just below the skin. This may not be a regular form of therapy, but it provides rapid onset of action. It can be prescribed for RLS because it is approved for Parkinson's disease and has been tested on a few people with RLS. Apomorphine may be used as an emergency medication if RLS symptoms occur unexpectedly.

Intravenous medications offer another advantage because they can be given when it is not possible to take medications by mouth. This is important after surgery or in some cases of serious illness. Some narcotics are already available in this format; dopaminergic medications may also be available. Another possible advantage of intravenous medications is that they bypass the barrier between the inside of the gut and the rest of the body. As mentioned earlier, iron can have a tough time getting into the body, and perhaps an even harder time getting into the brain. Intravenous iron is already being given to people with critical iron deficiency and those who are on dialysis. Early studies suggest that intravenous iron can provide a relatively long-term benefit for some people with RLS. Intravenous iron may even allow someone to stop taking other medications for RLS. Excess iron is toxic and can cause liver failure, perhaps even brain disease, and caution is warranted. The benefits and drawbacks of intravenous iron will be studied with great interest in coming years. We do not know what the final conclusion will be, but we are hopeful that intravenous iron will become a useful medication for many people with RLS.

Medications can also be delivered directly into the CSF in order to reach the brain directly. It is possible to gain access to the CSF by performing a spinal tap; however, it is also possible to put medication into the CSF through a tube. The advantage of this is that the medication goes straight into the brain. Usually this is not done as a one-time procedure, but rather a pump is placed to regularly send medication into the *intrathecal* space of the CSF. The pump can be placed under the skin near the bottom of the spine with a fine tube leading into the space. This has already been done in a few RLS patients. Narcotics can then be pumped in for pain relief. Dopaminergic drugs could also be adapted to this methodology. Besides the direct delivery to the brain, another advantage of this treatment is that small doses can be given. This may reduce the side effects that occur if a medication is given by mouth. This is a complicated therapy, but it may become a real option in the future for people with severe RLS.

What about surgery? One approach often used for pain and for multiple sclerosis is to place a stimulator over the spinal cord. This has been tried in a few people with RLS. How well this will work is unknown, but it may become another option for people with severe RLS. A procedure called deep brain stimulation (DBS) has become relatively standard treatment for advanced Parkinson's disease. Through a small hole in the skull, a thin stimulating electrode is placed in specific centers deep inside the brain (the thalamus, globus pallidus, or subthalamus). These centers or nuclei are thought to be involved in producing Parkinson's disease, and stimulating them often works to correct the motor problems experienced by people with this disease. Because Parkinson's is so debilitating, people are willing, often eager, to undergo this procedure, which can be quite beneficial. Few people with RLS want to have brain surgery, but those who have come to the end of the line and are not helped by medication may wish to try. One physician was caring for a man with Parkinson's disease who also had RLS. After surgery the patient's condition was improved, but so was his RLS! One group of movement disorder specialists has mentioned that they think DBS could work for RLS and that they would be willing to try this stimulation treatment for RLS.

What other treatments may come along somewhat further in the future? These are likely to come from the kinds of studies that are now being done to understand what causes RLS. To get some idea of what the future holds, we can look to science for answers.

THE SCIENCE OF RLS

The key role that Karl Ekbom played in teaching physicians about RLS cannot be diminished. He sent out the alarm and helped us recognize the problem that is RLS. But when it comes to a detailed understanding of what RLS is and how to treat it, almost everything has been learned in the last 10–15 years. The pace of discovery is likely to increase.

We are likely to learn several important things in the next 5–10 years. First, we are going to find genes for RLS. We already know there will not be a single gene for RLS; there may be a handful that are really important, and perhaps hundreds that have some role. We can expect that what has already happened in Parkinson's disease will happen in RLS. Only 9 years ago, the discovery of the first gene for Parkinson's was announced. The gene makes a protein called α-synuclein. Since then, more than a half dozen more genes have been found that cause some cases of Parkinson's disease. So we can expect that not one, but several genes for RLS will be known 5 years from now. Few people with Parkinson's have a mutation in the α-synuclein gene. This might seem disappointing, and the same situation may arise in RLS. But discovery of the α-synuclein gene also led to a better understanding of PD. Similarly, finding genes for RLS will help us understand what causes RLS, even if most people with RLS have none of the important mutant genes we discover.

What about finding the cause for RLS? In Chapter 3 the current understanding of the iron–dopamine connection in RLS was discussed. We do not yet know if this "connection" is the real key to understanding RLS, a part of the picture, or even a "red herring" that has put us off the real cause. Those of us in the field hope that the iron–dopamine connection is the real thing, because at least we will have made some steps in the right direction. In any case, in 5–10 years we should know whether the iron–dopamine connection is an important factor in causing RLS. But we may also find that some completely unexpected pathways are involved in RLS. Science is full of surprises. We can be cautiously optimistic that 10 years from now we will know as much about RLS, its genetics and causes, as is known today about Parkinson's disease.

FINAL WORDS

There may never be a gene therapy for RLS. There may never even be a cure for RLS, but it seems sure that the lives of people with RLS will be changed dramatically, and for the better, in coming decades. A major byproduct of the development of approved medications for RLS and the progress in understanding RLS will be the growing recognition of RLS by both the medical profession and the public. The problems that some people with RLS have had for years—if not decades—of being ignored, put off, or incorrectly treated by physicians who did not believe in RLS will be a thing of the past. RLS will become a routine part of the practice of medicine, known to every general practitioner. There will be effective ways to treat every degree of RLS. The public will understand that RLS is not a joke or a trivial affliction, but a sometimes serious problem that can ruin one's quality of life if it is not treated.

Rush Limbaugh made fun of RLS on his radio show. If he could live for one night as a severely affected RLS patient, he might find that other medical problems (such as his back problem or his profound hearing loss) are not nearly as bad as a night spent endlessly walking to ward off the "creepy-crawlies." He might recognize, as one patient did, that heart disease can be a problem, but RLS can be worse: although heart disease can kill you, you have to *live* with RLS. Maybe we should send him a copy of this book so he can educate himself and his radio audience.

Many people think the name of this disturbing disorder, *restless legs*, is not serious enough. Perhaps it should be changed, maybe to something snappy like *quiescogenic focal nocturnal akathisia*. Maybe someday it will be changed—once we understand the key to RLS, it may make sense to change the name to reflect that understanding. This is a standard procedure in naming medical disorders. On the other hand, maybe we should keep it. Why abandon a winner that has brought us so far?

Resources

ORGANIZATIONS

The RLS Foundation

819 Second Street, SW
Rochester, MN 55902-2985
rlsfoundation@rls.org
www.rls.org
Tel: 507-287-6465
Fax: 507-287-6312

The RLS Foundation is the best overall source of RLS information and help. Every RLS patient should join this nonprofit organization (only $25 per year). Membership includes the quarterly RLS newsletter *NightWalkers*, which contains up-to-date news about RLS, reviews of medical research articles, advice from RLS experts, a list of support groups, RLS stories from people and many other interesting topics. You also receive a free Medical Alert Card, set of chart stickers, and a medical bulletin that you can show to your physician.

The Foundation's Web site has a list of medical providers who are willing to treat RLS. You can also check out the latest RLS research projects and see if they need volunteers. The Web site has an active RLS discussion board and chat room. You can find a support group on their Web site or find out how to start your own support group.

Several different RLS Foundation publications (such as *RLS and Surgery, Living with RLS, Depression and RLS, Pregnancy and RLS, Children and RLS,* and the medical mulletin that reviews RLS treatment) are available on their Web site. The Foundation can mail them to you or you can download them yourself. Other articles can also be found on their Web site.

American Academy of Sleep Medicine (AASM)

One Westbrook Corporate Center, Suite 920
Westchester, IL 60154
www.aasmnet.org
Tel: 708-492-0930
Fax: 708-492-0943

The American Academy of Sleep Medicine is the premier organization devoted to the advancement of sleep medicine and sleep-related research. It also serves as the key resource for public and professional education on sleep disorders. As of 2006 it is comprised of close to 5000 individual members and more than 500 sleep center members.

The AASM's educational website is at www.sleepeducation.com (which also includes patient information and on-line forums) and individuals with sleep problems can locate the sleep center nearest to them at www.sleepcenters.org.

National Institutes of Health (NIH)

The NIH (www.nih.gov), a part of the U.S. Department of Health and Human Services, is the primary federal agency conducting and supporting medical research. Many other organizations make up the NIH, covering different health specialties. Three of these organizations offer valuable information on RLS:

National Institute of Neurological Disorders and Stroke (NINDS)

The NINDS Web site (www.ninds.nih.gov) contains a wealth of information on neurological disorders. The site contains a Restless Legs Syndrome Information Page (www.ninds.nih.gov/disorders/restless_

legs/restless_legs.htm#What_is) and a Restless Legs Syndrome Fact Sheet Page (www.ninds.nih.gov/disorders/restless_legs/vdetail_restless_legs.htm).

The National Heart, Lung, and Blood Institute (NHLBI)

NHLBI Information Center
P.O. Box 30105
Bethesda, MD 20824-0105
(301) 251-1222
(301) 251-1223 (fax)

The NHLBI (www.nhlbi.nih.gov/index.htm) has a sleep section (www.nhlbi.nih.gov/health/public/sleep/rls.htm) where you can download or order a free 4-page pamphlet *Fact Sheet on RLS*.

They also have another Web page (www.nhlbi.nih.gov/health/prof/sleep/rls_gde.htm) where you can download or order a free hard copy of this 16-page document called *Restless Legs Syndrome: Detection and Management in Primary Care*. This document would be helpful for your primary care physician.

The National Library of Medicine (NLM)

The NLM (www.nlm.nih.gov) is a great source of health information. It offers two areas of special interest to people with RLS:

1. Medline Plus (medlineplus.gov) contains information on drugs and over 700 health topics. They have a separate section on RLS (www.nlm.nih.gov/medlineplus/restlesslegs.html) that contains many interesting links to RLS topics.
2. PubMed (www.ncbi.nlm.nih.gov/entrez/query.fcgi?DB=pubmed) is a medical literature search service. Abstracts (summaries) of articles are free, but you may have to pay a small fee to obtain the full article. You may have to purchase some articles directly from the journal or publisher.

OTHER WEB SITES

The Southern California RLS Support Group

www.rlshelp.org contains detailed information about the drugs used for RLS and has pages of letters from people all over the world with medical replies from the first author of this book, Mark J. Buchfuhrer, MD.

The RLS Rebel Web site

rlsrebel.com is written by Jill Gunzel, aka the "RLS Rebel," and is a "must read" for all people with RLS. Jill has suffered from RLS for over 40 years and has a innovative approach for treating RLS. Included are many novel tricks to combat RLS symptoms.

WE MOVE

www.wemove.org contains a page (www.wemove.org/rls) that reviews RLS extensively, with detailed information about the treatment and drugs used for RLS.

Talk About Sleep

www.talkaboutsleep.com covers many sleep topics, including RLS. It also has chat rooms and message boards on RLS/PLMD topics.

Bandolier Web site

Bandolier is a publishing company that has print and Internet (www.jr2.ox.ac.uk/bandolier) versions of many medical articles. By typing RLS in its search box, you will find reviews of 36 articles on RLS.

Johns Hopkins Center for RLS

www.neuro.jhmi.edu/rls has educational and research information on RLS. Johns Hopkins is the most active center doing research on the role of dopamine and iron in RLS.

National Sleep Foundation

www.sleepfoundation.org http://www.sleepfoundation.orghas a wealth of sleep information and an RLS article reviewed by Richard Allen, PhD and Merrill M. Mitler, PhD.

Mayo Clinic Proceedings Journal

By entering the journal's Web site (www.mayoclinicproceedings.com) you can click on *Past Issues* and then on *July 2004* to view or download a free copy of the article "An Algorithm for the Management of Restless Legs Syndrome." This article reviews the management of RLS and presents guidelines for treating intermittent, daily, and refractory RLS. Bring a copy of this article to your physician if he or she needs help managing your RLS.

RLS MEESSAGE/BULLETIN BOARDS, FORUMS, AND CHAT ROOMS

These are Internet meeting places where people with RLS can contact and discuss RLS with others who have similar problems. You can leave messages (called posts) about almost any RLS topic and usually get answers or opinions from others. The chat rooms do much the same thing, but occur immediately as participants type in their responses. Some of these services require you to become a member and get a password (this is a free service) before you can participate.

The RLS Foundation's chat room and bulletin board

www.rls.org has some excellent discussion groups about all aspects of RLS. It is a active board with lots of current posts. A chat room is also available.

Cyberspace RLS Support Group

health.groups.yahoo.com/group/rlssupport is a discussion list for RLS/PLMD sufferers. Topics include RLS treatments, medications, and alternative therapies.

The We Move Discussion Forum

www.wemove.org runs this active board.

RLS_PLMD at Yahoo groups

health.groups.yahoo.com/group/RLS_PLMD is an e-mail list support group for people with active or severe restless legs syndrome and/or periodic limb movement disorder. RLS_PLMD at Yahoo groups designed their site specifically for people who have found no benefit from herbs, supplements, over-the-counter remedies, or do-it-yourself home treatments and would rather not deal with lots of e-mails pertaining to their use. These subjects are off-topic for this group and should be discussed elsewhere. This group is moderately active.

Talk About Sleep

www.talkaboutsleep.com has message boards for many sleep topics including RLS/PLMD. It has a moderate amount of posts for RLS/PLMD. It also has periodic scheduled chat times on RLS/PLMD.

Sleep Net

www.sleepnet.com/rls/rlsinf.html has message boards for many sleep topics, including RLS/PLMD, with a moderate amount of posts.

HealthBoard.com

www.healthboards.com has message boards for many health-related problems, including RLS. It has moderate activity.

Brain Talk Communities

brain.hastypastry.net/forums has forums for many neurological disorders, including RLS. The RLS discussion forum is mild to moderately active.

SUPPORT GROUPS

All of the American and Canadian support groups are associated with the RLS Foundation. You can find a complete list of these groups on the RLS Foundation's Web site (www.rls.org) or in their quarterly newsletter, *NightWalkers*. Additionally, several independent international support groups work in cooperation with the RLS Foundation.

PAMPHLETS

The following pamphlets can be downloaded from www.rls.org or ordered directly from the RLS Foundation:

> *Living with RLS*
> *Surgery and RLS*
> *Depression and RLS*
> *Pregnancy and RLS*
> *Children and RLS*
> *Medical Bulletin* (reviews RLS treatment)
> *RLS Scientific Bulletin* (reviews RLS research and new treatments)
> *RLS: Detection & Management in Primary Care* (NIH document)
> *Understanding & Diagnosing RLS* (video)

RLS information can be downloaded from www.sleepeducation.com, an educational website by the American Academy of Sleep Medicine.

The National Heart, Lung, and Blood Institute (NHLBI)

The following pamphlets can be downloaded from http://www.nhlbi.nih.gov/health/public/sleep/rls.htm or ordered directly:

Facts about RLS (4-page pamphlet)
RLS: Detection & Management in Primary Care (16-page pamphlet)

BOOKS ON RLS

Chaudhuri, K. Ray, Odin, P., Olanow, C W. *Restless Legs Syndrome*. Taylor & Francis, New York, 2004.

This is the first professional-level book written on RLS. Written by a panel of experts, *Restless Legs Syndrome* focuses on the diagnosis and management of RLS. The authors discuss the epidemiology of RLS, pathophysiology, clinical associations, and clinical features. They explore how to diagnose the many different types of people who present with this disorder. It includes discussions of the wide range of treatment options available in order to give clinicians the information they need to formulate appropriate pharmacological or nonpharmacological therapeutic regimens.

Cunningham, Chet. *Stopping Restless Leg Syndrome*. United Research Publishers, Encinitas, CA 2000.

This book was written by an author who specializes in consumer-focused health books.

Gunzel, Jill. *Restless Legs Syndrome: The RLS Rebel's Survival Guide*. Wheatmark, Inc., Tucson, AZ, 2006.

This book describes the RLS Rebel Program, an outline which helps RLSers (people with RLS) organize their fight against RLS and achieve maximize results from any combination of RLS treatments. When treatments include use of prescription drugs, the RLS Rebel Program becomes the ultimate complementary medicine approach to RLS. The book includes six steps for reducing aggravating variables, suggestions for developing and using a "bag of tricks approach," tips for better communication with medical professionals, advice to supporters of RLSers, suggestions for using the RLS Rebel Program with children, and information about dealing with RLS on long trips and in other special situations.

Ondo, William G. *Restless Leg Syndrome (Neurological Disease and Therapy)*. Informa Healthcare/Taylor & Francis, New York, 2006.

The book, edited by William Ondo, is an authoritative and comprehensive guide on RLS. It examines the pathogenesis, diagnosis, and treatment the disorder. Ranging from basic science to therapeutics, *Restless Leg Syndrome* analyzes the many new and emerging medications impacting the management of this disorder and strives to address the explosion of research in the field.

Wilson, Virginia N. (Walters, A. S., ed.) *Sleep Thief, Restless Legs Syndrome*. Galaxy Books Inc., Orange Park, FL, 1996.

This is the first book on RLS. Written by one of the founders of the RLS Foundation, and contains both a layperson's perspective and professional essays from a variety of medical experts.

Yoakum, Robert. *Restless Legs Syndrome: Relief and Hope for Sleepless Victims of a Hidden Epidemic*. Simon & Schuster, New York, 2006.

This book details the reality of RLS and its problems, as well as reviewing coping, therapy, and the science of RLS. The book brings alive the real suffering of the severe patient with RLS and includes a multitude of individual testimonies. The author is a former member of the Board of Directors of the RLS Foundation and author of the historical article on RLS published in *Modern Maturity* in 1994. He prepared this volume in consultation with a variety of RLS experts, including members of the RLSF Medical Advisory board.

The Official Patient's Sourcebook on Restless Leg Syndrome. Icon Health Publications, San Diego, CA, 2002.

This draws from public, academic, government, and peer-reviewed research; provides guidance on how to obtain free-of-charge, primary research results as well as more detailed information via the Internet. E-book and electronic versions of this sourcebook are fully interactive with each of the Internet sites mentioned.

BOOKS ON RELATIONSHIPS

Atwood, Nina. *Soul Talk: Powerful, Positive Communication for a Loving Partnership.* Sourcebooks, Naperville, IL, 2003.

Donoghue, Paul J., Siegel, Mary E. *Are You Really Listening? Keys to Successful Communication.* Sorin Books, Notre Dame, IN, 2005.

Hamburg, Sam R. *Will Our Love Last: A Couple's Road Map.* Scribner, New York, 200.

McKay, Matthew, Fanning, Patrick, Paleg, Kim. *Couple Skills: Making Your Relationship Work.* New Harbinger Publications, Oakland, CA, 1994.

Tannen, Deborah. *You Just Don't Understand.* Harper Collins, New York, 2001.

MEDICAL ALERT CARDS

There are three sources for RLS medical alert cards:

1. The RLS Foundation (www.rls.org), which gives them out free as part of membership.

2. The Southern California RLS Support Group (www.rlshelp.org). Download a copy for free and print it on your own home printer. Cardstock copies available for free from this group if you cannot download them. To have one mailed, please send a self-addressed, stamped envelope (SASE) to:

   Janis Lopes
   125 East Mayfair Avenue
   Orange, CA 92867

   Please add additional postage for each request of more than nine cards.

3. The Greater San Antonio RLS Support Group (www.legsmove.org/med-card.htm) sells cards for $2.00 for 10 cards.

INFORMATION FOR PREGNANT OR BREASTFEEDING WOMEN

www.motherisk.org

www.perinatology.com
http://orpheus.ucsd.edu/ctis/

INSURANCE

For those people with RLS who find themselves unable to get insurance, some resources are available. The Health Assistance Partnership was established to address the needs of the nation's consumer health assistance programs. These programs serve Medicaid and Medicare beneficiaries, privately insured consumers, and the uninsured. Their Web site has a wealth of information on obtaining insurance. You can also contact them at the address below.

Health Assistance Partnership

1201 New York Avenue NW, Suite 1100
Washington, DC 20005
202-737-6340
www.healthassistancepartnership.org

The AARP (www.aarp.org) also has excellent resources for those people with RLS in the Medicare gap years, from ages 50–65. Their Web site reviews all the various insurance options and has many helpful pointers on how to obtain insurance. For those people who lose their health insurance upon losing their job or after a divorce, this site has a complete description of COBRA (Consolidated Omnibus Budget Reconciliation Act) insurance coverage.

People without insurance, who must pay cash, must look for other options. Many drug companies have drug assistance plans that provide their drugs free or at much reduced costs to people without insurance. Some of these plans do not require proof of financial need. Another option is to buy drugs outside of the U.S. at a lower cost.

Glossary

Addiction: Addiction is a primary, chronic, neurobiologic disease, with genetic, psychosocial, and environmental factors influencing its development and manifestations. It is characterized by behaviors that include one or more of the following: impaired control over drug use, compulsive use, continued use despite harm, and craving.

Agonist: A drug capable of combining with receptors to initiate drug actions. An example is a dopamine drug acting on the dopamine receptors to cause actions similar to the effect of the body's own dopamine.

Akithisea: A medical condition manifested by a sense of inner restlessness with an inability to remain still or motionless. It occurs most often as a side effect of the drugs used to treat schizophrenia and other psychoses, antinausea drugs, or when the drugs used to treat Parkinson's disease are withdrawn. Unlike RLS, akathisia can occur at any time of the day, usually only when the patient is sitting but not when lying down, and the restlessness is generalized and not located only in a limb.

Algorithm: A step-by-step protocol for management of a health care problem.

Antagonist: A drug that has binds to a receptor but does not activate the receptor. The drug blocks the affect of other drugs or chemicals produced by the body that normally bind and activate these receptors.

Apnea: The cessation or near complete cessation (over 70 percent reduction) or airflow for a minimum of 10 seconds.

Augmentation: A worsening of RLS symptoms that occurs after starting a drug to treat RLS (this may only occur with dopaminergic drugs). Symptoms may occur earlier in the day, shift to body parts other than the legs, become more intense or begin after a shorter period of rest.

Benzodiazepines: Sedative, hypnotic or antianxiety drugs that are related to Valium® (diazepam). Although most benzodiazepines are marketed for either their sedative or hypnotic effect (but not both), they are usually effective as sleeping or antianxiety drugs.

Chromosome: A chromosome (normally 22 pairs in humans) is a long, continuous piece of DNA, which contains many genes and is found in the nucleus of the body's cells. Every chromosome is made up of two paired strands of DNA, some part of which "codes" for genes, and some of which has other functions (perhaps unknown) or even no clear function.

Circadian: Relating to biologic variations or rhythms with a cycle of about 24 hours.

Counterstimulation: Using a stimulus (such as a sensory input from hot or cold water) to distract from another usually bothersome sensation (such as pain or RLS).

Dependence: See Physical and Psychological Dependence.

Dopamine agonist: A drug that acts upon the dopamine receptors to cause the same effect as the body's own dopamine. This includes bromocriptine (Parlodel®), pergolide (Permax®), cabergoline (Dostinex®), pramipexole (Mirapex®) ropinirole (Requip®), apomorphine (Apokyn"), and rotigotine.

Dopamine: A brain neurotransmitter important for motor function and the manner in which we experience reward behavior as pleasurable. Dopamine is important in Parkinson's disease (where it is decreased due to the loss of dopamine containing brain cells) and in RLS (where it is present but does not function normally).

Dopaminergic: Relating to nerve cells or fibers that employ dopamine as their neurotransmitter. Drugs that act similar to dopamine on the dopamine system are called dopaminergic drugs.

Drug holiday: Stopping a drug for a short time (up to several weeks) to reestablish effectiveness. Some drugs (such as dopamine agonists and opioids) may become less effective due to tolerance and can have effectiveness restored after a drug holiday.

Dysesthesia: A disagreeable or abnormal sensation.

Echocardiogram: Ultrasound evaluation of the heart (used to look for heart valve damage among other problems).

Epidemiology: The study of the distribution and determinants of disease in human populations and the application of this study to control health problems.

Ergot alkaloid–derived dopamine agonist: A dopamine agonist that is created from ergot alkaloids (a chemical produced by a fungus that infects rye and other plants). This includes bromocriptine (Parlodel®), pergolide (Permax®), cabergoline (Dostinex®).

Ferritin: A protein that forms a complex to transport and store iron in the body. The blood ferritin level is a more accurate estimate of body iron stores than serum iron levels. However, ferritin is also an acute phase reactant. This means it increases with any sudden illness and so cannot be accurately measured if someone is sick, as with the flu or arthritis.

Formulary: A list of drugs that insurance companies cover with different copayments.

Half-life: The time required for one-half the amount of a substance (drug) to be lost through biologic processes (metabolized and/or excreted).

Hemochromatosis: A disorder of iron metabolism characterized by excessive absorption of ingested iron, saturation of iron-binding protein, and deposition of iron in tissues, particularly in the liver, pancreas, and skin; cirrhosis of the liver, diabetes (bronze diabetes), bronze pigmentation of the skin, and, eventually heart failure may occur; also can result from administration of large amounts of iron orally, by injection, or in forms of blood transfusion therapy.

Hypersomnia: Excessive sleepiness.

Hypnotic: An agent that promotes sleep; also called *sleeping pills.*

Hypopnea: Partial reduction (more than 30 percent but not more than 70 percent) in airflow for a minimum of 10 seconds.

Idiopathic: Disease of unknown cause or origin.

Maintenance of Wakefulness Test (MWT): A test in which subjects are instructed to stay awake while relaxed in a darkened room. The amount of time before falling asleep is considered an indication of the ability to stay awake.

Multiple Sleep Latency Test (MSLT): A test with four to five naps spaced at 2-hour intervals performed the morning and afternoon. This may be done after a nighttime sleep study. The MSLT is used to asses the level of daytime sleepiness.

Narcolepsy: A sleep disorder that usually appears in young adulthood consisting of recurring episodes of irresistible sleep during the day and often disrupted nocturnal sleep. In its complete form, there may be vivid hallucinations when falling asleep and waking and sudden attacks of weakness, called *cataplexy.* These attacks can be provoked by strong emotion, such as laughter or fear.

Narcotic: Pain-killing drugs, synthetic or naturally occurring, with effects similar to those of opium and opium derivatives. Also called opioids or opiates.

Neuroleptic: Drugs treat psychotic conditions such as schizophrenia.

Neuropathy: A disorder of one or more of the nerves outside the central nervous system (the brain and spinal cord). Peripheral neuropathy applies to a disorder affecting nerves such as those going to the arms or, most commonly, the legs.

Neurotransmitter: Any specific chemical agent released by a nerve cell, upon excitation, that crosses to receiving side of another nerve cell (across the synapse) to signal (by stimulating or inhibiting) the other nerve cell. These are the chemicals that nerve cells use to communicate with one another.

Nocturnal myoclonus: Original term for Periodic Limb Movements. This term is outdated and no longer used.

Non–ergot-derived dopamine agonist: A dopamine agonist that is not derived from ergot alkaloids (a chemical produced by a fungus that infects rye and other plants). This includes pramipexole (Mirapex®) and ropinirole (Requip®), and rotigotine.

Off-label: This is the practice of prescribing drugs for a purpose outside the scope of the drug's approved (in the U.S., approved by the FDA) label or indication. Off-label use does not mean the drug is forbidden, only that the FDA has not certified the drug for use in that specific condition.

Opioids: Painkiller medications that are derived from or chemically related to opium; also called *narcotics*.

Paresthesia: An abnormal skin sensation, such as burning, prickling, itching, or tingling.

Peripheral neuropathy: A disorder affecting nerves of the peripheral nervous system such as those going to the arms or, most commonly, the legs. The damage to the nerves results in abnormal sensations (numbess, pins and needles, etc.) or weakness to the affected area.

Periodic Limb Movement Disorder (PLMD): A medical disorder resulting from a significant frequency of PLMS during sleep with a related clinical complaint such as daytime sleepiness. The PLMS cannot be due to another disorder (such as sleep apnea, narcolepsy or RLS). Therefore, people with RLS cannot have PLMD.

Periodic Limb Movement(s) (PLMS): One or more leg movement in a series of rhythmic repetitive leg movements, often having extension of the big toe, dorsiflexion of the ankle with or without flexion of the knee and hip occurring in wake or sleep. The movement can also occur in the arms. This term can also be used as the plural form for many limb movements.

Physical dependence: A state of adaptation that often includes tolerance and is manifested by a drug class specific withdrawal syndrome that can be produced by abrupt cessation, rapid dose reduction, decreasing blood level of the drug, and/or administration of an antagonist. Physical dependence is a purely bodily function and may not include addiction or psychological dependence, which are disorders or behavioral conditions.

Placebo: Sugar pill, or sham, therapy used for the control group during research trials of treatments.

Polysomnogram: A sleep study with multiple monitoring electrodes that record various activities of sleep (brain waves, breathing, oxygen level, pulse, etc.). This test is used to diagnose sleep disorders such as sleep apnea, narcolepsy, or PLMD.

Postsynaptic terminal: The part of a nerve cell (or nonnerve cells such as muscle or gland cells) that contains receptors for a neurotransmitter chemical that has been released across a synapse by the presynaptic terminal of a nerve.

Presynaptic terminal: The part of a nerve cell that releases a neurotransmitter chemical that crosses a synapse to attach to the receptors on the postsynaptic terminal of another nerve cell (or nonnerve cells such as muscle or gland cells).

Psychological dependence: The result of repeated consumption of a drug that produces psychological but no physical dependence. The psychological dependence produces a desire (not a compulsion) to continue taking drugs for the sense of improved well-being.

Psychomotor retardation: A slowing of activities that require mental and physical effort. Speech, thoughts, and movements are slow. There is reduced spontaneous movement and a general lack of alacrity. This can be seen in depression or dementia.

Rebound: A worsening of RLS symptoms several hours after taking a dose of medication (usually a dopamine type drug) to treat RLS. This is due to the short half-life of a medication that does not last long enough to treat RLS symptoms that occur after its therapeutic effect has worn off.

Refractory: Resistant to treatment.

Sedative: A drug that reduces anxiety by exerting a calming effect.

Serum: The fluid part of blood (with the blood cells and clotting factors removed). Most lab values (such as iron and ferritin levels) are reported as serum levels.

Sleep apnea: A sleep disorder caused by recurrent interruptions of breathing during sleep. Usually refers to obstructive sleep apnea that is caused by obstruction of the airway during sleep often accompanied with loud snoring and daytime sleepiness.

Sleep hygiene: A set of guidelines for improving sleep that includes avoiding behaviors and substances that disturb sleep.

Substantia nigra: Portion of the midbrain thought to be involved in certain aspects of movement and attention. The substantia nigra is one of the major areas in the brain that contains dopamine, which is depleted in Parkinson's disease.

Synapse: A synapse is a specialized junction through which cells of the nervous system signal to one another (using signaling chemicals known as neurotransmitters) and to nonnerve cells such as muscles or glands.

Taper: Slowly stop the use of a drug by gradually decreasing the dose over several days or weeks.

Titrate: Increase the dose of a drug slowly until it becomes effective. This is used to find the lowest effective dose while avoiding the greater side effects that might come with higher doses.

Tolerance: A decrease over time in effect of a drug on a person that usually requires the person to take a larger dose to maintain the original response.

Transferrin receptor: Receptor on the surface of cells that binds transferrin (when loaded with iron). Transferrin receptor levels increase to help facilitate iron delivery into the body's cells. Transferrin receptor levels are one of the most accurate measures of the body's iron stores, because they do not vary with other disease states.

Transferrin: This protein carries iron in the blood and delivers it to cells in the body. When transferrin loaded with iron encounters a transferrin receptor on the surface of a cell, it binds to it and is consequently transported into the cell. Transferrin levels increase in iron deficiency anemia. However, the amount of iron attached to transferrin (percent iron saturation) is decreased in iron deficiency anemia and increased in hemochromatosis.

Tyrosine hydroxylase: A key enzyme needed to produce dopamine in the body. This enzyme needs iron to be active and may cause a bottleneck in the production of dopamine when iron levels are low.

List of Abbreviations

ADHD—attention deficit–hyperactivity disorder (also called ADD for attention deficit disorder).

CAM—complementary and alternative medicine.

CPAP—continuous positive airway pressure. A CPAP machine is an air pump that delivers air under pressure to the airways by a mask or nasal pillows. The air pressure forces the collapsed airway to open and prevents apnea.

CSF—cerebrospinal fluid. The fluid that surrounds the brain and spinal column.

CT—computed tomography scan. A three-dimensional X-ray that requires the patient to enter into the tunnel or tube of a CT scanner.

DBS—deep brain stimulation.

EEG—electroencephalography or the electrical recording of brain waves.

EEOC—Equal Employment Opportunity Commission.

EMG—electromyography or the electrical recording of muscle activity.

ER—emergency room.

ESRD—end-stage renal disease. This term applies to people with complete kidney failure who usually need dialysis.

FDA—U.S. Food and Drug Administration.

HMO—health maintenance organization.

IRLS—International Restless Legs Syndrome Study Group rating scale; the accepted rating scale for RLS that is used in research studies.

IRLSSG—International Restless Legs Syndrome Study Group.

MRI—magnetic resonance imaging. An MRI scan requires the patient enter a tube (although some open MRI scanners are available), but does not use radiation as an imaging source but rather magnetic resonance to create a three-dimensional image of the body part that it examines.

MSLT—multiple sleep latency test. Four to five nap studies performed through the morning and afternoon, usually after a nighttime sleep study. The patient is asked to try to go to sleep. The MSLT is used to asses the level of daytime sleepiness.

MWT—maintenance of wakefulness test. A test in which subjects are instructed to stay awake while relaxed in a darkened room. The amount of time taken to fall asleep is considered an indication of the ability to stay awake.

NCCAM—National Center for Complementary and Alternative Medicine.

NCSDR—National Center for Sleep Disorders Research. This center is a part of the NHLBI.

NHLBI—National Heart, Blood, and Lung Institute.

NIH—National Institutes of Health.

NREM sleep—non–rapid-eye-movement sleep or sleep other than dreaming sleep. There are four stages of NREM sleep from stage 1 sleep (very light sleep) to stages 3 and 4 (very deep sleep).

OHA—Office of Hearings and Appeals.

OSA—obstructive sleep apnea.

PD—Parkinson's disease.

PDR—*Physicians' Desk Reference*, the drug book that physicians use to look up information on the drugs that they prescribe.

PET—positron emission tomography. The PET scan is a nuclear medicine imaging technique which produces a three-dimensional image or map of functional processes in the body using radioactive tracers.

PLM—periodic limb movement(s). One or more leg movement in a series of rhythmic repetitive leg movements manifested by extension of the big toe, dorsiflexion of the ankle with or without flexion of the knee and hip occurring in wake or sleep. The movement can also occur in the arms. This term can also be used as the plural form for many limb movements.

PLMA—periodic limb movement(s) with arousals. These are leg movements that occur during sleep and result in a shift from deeper to lighter sleep.

PLMAI—periodic limb movement arousal index. The number of PLMS associated with an arousal per hour of sleep.

PLMD—periodic limb movement disorder. A medical disorder resulting from a significant frequency of PLMS during sleep with a related clinical complaint such as daytime sleepiness. The PLMS cannot be due to another disorder (such as sleep apnea, narcolepsy, or RLS).

PLMI—periodic limb movement index. The number of PLM per hour. Usually refers to the number of PLMS per each hour of sleep.

PLMS—periodic limb movement(s) in sleep. One or more PLM that occur during sleep. Usually used in the plural form referring to all the leg movements that occur during sleep or to the condition of having these leg movements during sleep.

PLMW—periodic limb movement(s) during wakefulness. One or more PLM that occur while the patient is awake. Usually used in the plural form.

PSG—polysomnogram or sleep study.

REM sleep—rapid-eye-movement sleep or dreaming sleep.

RLS—restless legs syndrome.

RLSF—RLS Foundation.

SIT—suggested immobilization test. This test is used to examine the effect of drugs on RLS symptoms or PLM by having the subject sit while instructed not to move for a period of time (usually 40 minutes to an hour).

SNRI—serotonin- and norepinephrine-reuptake inhibitor. These drugs are usually used to fight depression, but may aggravate RLS. Also called SSNRI.

SRBD—sleep-related breathing disorder. SRBD refers to any disturbance of breathing during sleep, such as obstructive and nonobstructive sleep apnea, hypopnea, and upper airway resistance syndrome.

SSA—Social Security Administration.

SSD—Social Security disability insurance.

SSI —Supplemental Security Income.

SSNRI—selective serotonin- and norepinephrine-reuptake inhibitor. These drugs are usually used to fight depression, but may aggravate RLS. Also called SNRI.

SSRI—selective serotonin-reuptake inhibitor. These drugs are usually used to fight depression, but may aggravate RLS.

TCA—tricyclic antidepressant. This includes the older antidepressant drugs such as amitriptyline (Elavil).

UARS—upper airway resistance syndrome. This condition is usually associated with loud snoring. Breathing is not blocked or even reduced (as with sleep apnea or hypopnea), but the person makes a greater effort to breathe against increased resistance, which results in snoring.

Index

NOTE: *Boldface numbers indicate illustrations; t indicates a table.*

Made in the USA
Monee, IL
17 July 2021